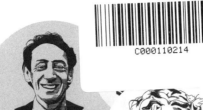

THE LITTLE BOOK OF

QUEER ICONS

SAMUEL ALEXANDER

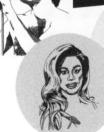

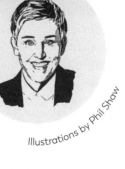

Illustrations by Phil Shaw

summersdale

THE LITTLE BOOK OF QUEER ICONS

Illustrations by Phil Shaw, 2018

An Hachette UK Company
www.hachette.co.uk

Summersdale Publishers Ltd
Part of Octopus Publishing Group Limited
Carmelite House
50 Victoria Embankment
LONDON
EC4Y 0DZ
UK

www.summersdale.com

Printed and bound in Malta

ISBN: 978-1-78685-777-4

CONTENTS

INTRODUCTION

Within these pages you will find many queer icons who have helped shape the world for queer people today. Not every story is a happy one – the fight for LGBTQ civil rights has been a long one and continues to this day. Along the way, we, as a community, have experienced tragic losses. It is important not to forget the stories of those who fought for queer liberation, because these people used their queer superpowers to make our lives better.

When asked which superpower you would rather have, it is not uncommon to hear the answer "invisibility". I have been guilty of giving that answer myself. For an anxious queer boy, having the option to hide away from a cruel world sounded like a dream come true. But in writing this book I have learned, as I hope you will too, that the strongest and most useful superpower for any queer person is not invisibility, but visibility.

The people in this book have all lived their lives as unapologetically queerly as they wanted to. From fighting for the rights of the LGBTQ community, to sharing their experiences and validating queer lives, they have been as visible as possible with their queer identities. They have raised their voices in solidarity with a community that still faces daily prejudice and oppression, and defiantly lived their truth.

Invisibility is safe, but it is lonely. Invisibility does not inspire change, but visibility demands it. In writing this book I have come to realize this and I truly believe it. We live in a world that is changing all the time and for every act of tolerance, intolerance is only ever a few steps behind. We have to be visible as the people we are.

We all have the power to inspire change, however small that change may be. Be unapologetic in your queerness, live your truth and change the world.

I hope these words, and the stories and experiences within, inspire you as they have me.

Be visible.

Samuel Alexander, 2018

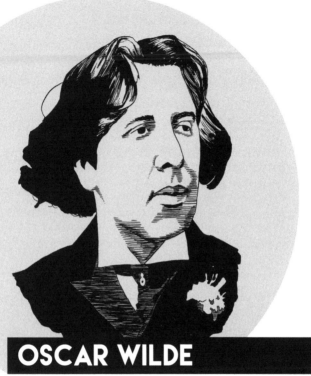

OSCAR WILDE

1854–1900

SUPERPOWERS

Flamboyant, bravely queer poet, writer, star pupil, academic.

THEIR INCREDIBLE STORY

The brilliant Irish writer and poet Oscar Wilde brought *The Picture of Dorian Gray* and *The Importance of Being Earnest* to life, although sadly his own story ended in tragedy.

Wilde studied classics at Trinity College Dublin in 1871 before moving on to Oxford's Magdalen College. While studying, Wilde developed an interest in Greek literature, and he would later become interested in the Aesthetic and Decadent movements. He was always a star pupil, graduating with high grades from both institutions. Wilde became well known for his stories, poems and plays, but he also wrote reviews of theatre and literature for *The Woman's World* magazine – of which he was editor from 1887 to 1889 – as well as many essays and articles for other magazines, which frequently proved controversial in their content.

When passages from *The Picture of Dorian Gray* were published in *Lippincott's Monthly Magazine* in 1890, the novel was heavily criticized for its homosexual allusions. When the book was published in 1891, Wilde felt forced to remove portions of text to avoid further allegations.

In 1895, Wilde found himself embroiled in a legal feud with the Marquess of Queensberry. In 1891, Wilde had begun a relationship with Lord Alfred Douglas, Queensberry's son, which led to Queensberry publicly accusing Wilde of sodomy. Wilde initiated a prosecution against Queensberry for criminal libel, but Queensberry avoided the charges when it became clear he could prove his allegations against Wilde. Wilde's private life became the subject of controversy and investigation, and the content of his writings – both public and private – were used as evidence against him.

A warrant was issued for Wilde's arrest – he was charged with "gross indecency" – and he was incarcerated in 1895. He spent his time in prison writing a long letter to Douglas, reflecting on his career and – sometimes scathingly – on their relationship. Wilde was not allowed to send the letter, but was permitted to carry it with him upon his release in 1897. After his release and before his exile to France, Wilde was briefly reunited with Douglas. They were forced to separate soon after, as their families threatened to cut them off financially if their relationship continued.

Wilde spent his final years in Paris in impoverished exile, writing letters calling for penal reform after suffering harsh treatment in prison, before his early death from meningitis in 1900. His former lover and dear friend, Robert Ross, was by his side in his final moments. Wilde's burial took place just outside Paris at Cimetière de Bagneux, but he was moved to Père Lachaise several years later, to a tomb built by sculptor Sir Jacob Epstein and commissioned by Ross.

Wilde was pardoned more than 100 years after his death, under the Alan Turing Law (see p.20).

THEIR AWESOME ACHIEVEMENTS

➜ Wrote many iconic stories, poems and plays. *The Picture of Dorian Gray* is one of his most famous literary works, a novel well known for its subtle queer themes.

➜ Wrote a 50,000-word letter, entitled *De Profundis*, while in prison, which he kept with him until he was released. The letter was addressed to his lover, Lord Alfred Douglas. The letter was entrusted to and published by Robert Ross after Wilde's death.

➜ Paved the way for queer rights in the arts, with his literary works brimming over with suggestion and subtle queer themes. They may seem tame by today's queer literary standards because Wilde was aware of the need to hide his sexuality. Despite this, he never expressed any shame in his sexuality.

➜ His legacy reminds us of the persecution faced by the LGBTQ community in Britain before the queer rights liberations of later years, and of the struggles still faced by the queer community in countries where LGBTQ rights are oppressed.

"BE YOURSELF; EVERYONE ELSE IS ALREADY TAKEN."

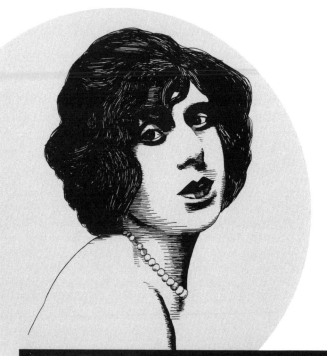

LILI ELBE

1882–1931

SUPERPOWERS

Sex-reassignment pioneer, painter, transgender woman, muse.

THEIR INCREDIBLE STORY

Lili Elbe was a Danish painter and transgender woman, and one of the first known people in the world to undergo sex-reassignment surgery.

Elbe studied at the Royal Danish Academy of Fine Arts, where she met Gerda Gottlieb, who would later become Elbe's wife. When a model failed to show for one of Gottlieb's paintings, Gottlieb's friend Anna Larson suggested that Elbe sit for the painting instead. Elbe found comfort in donning women's clothes for the role, and Larson remarked on how well the clothing suited Elbe, giving her the name Lili.

Elbe would soon begin to dress as a woman in public, encouraged by Gottlieb who would identify herself publicly as her sister. An internal struggle was happening at this time within Elbe, who felt like two people trapped in one body – a loving partner, Einar Wegener (Elbe's name prior to adopting Lili), and a carefree Lili, who desired to carry a child. People close to Elbe began to wonder whether Lili was an act or not, as Elbe seemed much more comfortable presenting as a woman. Elbe confided in Gottlieb that she felt she had always been Lili, and that Einar had gone.

They moved to Paris together in 1912, escaping the scrutiny of their peers in Denmark. Elbe was safe to start anew, identifying as a woman from the moment they arrived. However, she experienced discomfort in her body, which did not reflect her gender identity.

She became depressed and, without any resources on transgender issues, with no one to talk to and lacking the language to discuss transgender issues even if this hadn't been the case, she became suicidal – until she met German doctor Magnus Hirschfeld.

Hirschfeld opened the German Institute for Sexual Science in 1919, and became the first doctor to study transgender lives. After their meeting, Elbe underwent years of experimental surgery to change her body to match her gender identity – and this laid the groundwork for what is now known as gender-reassignment surgery. The initial surgery was conducted by Hirschfeld himself, who started with the removal of the male genitalia. Other surgeries were conducted by Kurt Warnekros, a doctor at the Dresden Municipal Women's Clinic, who had a focus on implanting female sex organs. Sadly, documentation of Elbe's transition was destroyed by the Nazis in 1933, so the finer details have been lost. But we do know that the fourth and final part of Elbe's surgery led to her death when a transplanted uterus was rejected.

Gottlieb remained supportive of Elbe throughout, allowing her the distance to be Lili independently, even after the King of Denmark dissolved their marriage. Danish law at the time did not recognize marriage between two women – though, more progressively, the law did recognize Elbe's identity as a woman. In 1933, the book *Man into Woman* was published, comprising diary entries and writings left behind by Elbe, in accordance with her last wishes. The book gave an account of Elbe's life and was one of the first widely available books about a transgender person's life.

THEIR AWESOME ACHIEVEMENTS

→ Winner of the Neuhausen prize for paintings displayed at the Vejle Art Museum, Denmark and Salon d'Automne, Paris, 1907.

→ The first recognized transgender person to undergo gender-reassignment surgery.

→ Became a pioneer in sex-reassignment, willingly put her own body at risk to develop and understand surgeries that are now practised successfully.

→ Proved that one's body isn't the sole determining factor in gender and that, if a person chooses, they can alter their body to match their gender identity.

"I CANNOT DENY, STRANGE AS IT MAY SOUND, THAT I ENJOYED MYSELF IN THIS DISGUISE. I LIKED THE FEEL OF SOFT WOMEN'S CLOTHING. I FELT VERY MUCH AT HOME IN THEM FROM THE FIRST MOMENT."

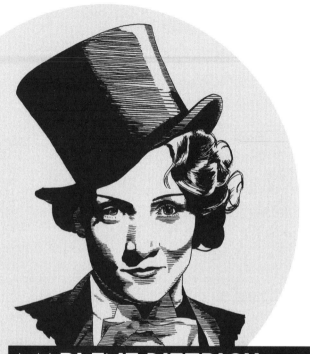

MARLENE DIETRICH

1901–92

SUPERPOWERS

*Bisexual goddess, humanitarian,
actress, androgynous and proud.*

THEIR INCREDIBLE STORY

German actress Marlene Dietrich was famed for her beauty, her film roles and her many lovers. However, she is also remembered for her anti-Nazi stance and humanitarian efforts. She also happened to be openly bisexual.

In 1929, Dietrich starred in Germany's first non-silent film, *Der Blaue Engel* (*The Blue Angel*), proving her talents as both an actor and singer with the role. Dietrich then made her move to Hollywood, making her mark as a femme fatale of the silver screen.

Hollywood was both welcoming and wary of Dietrich and it is thought that she never fully integrated. Her accent had allure which, combined with her looks, gave her performances an added touch of intrigue. However, she was always seen as "foreign", particularly in the political climate of the time. Nevertheless, Dietrich starred in many Hollywood roles.

During World War Two, Dietrich was very vocal in her opposition to the Nazi Party and anti-Semitism, saying she felt "abandoned" by Germany. She entertained US troops on the front line and took part in humanitarian efforts, housing both German and French exiles and fighting for their right to US citizenship. Later, Dietrich was honoured by the American and French governments with the Medal of Freedom and Légion d'Honneur respectively for her efforts.

Dietrich was iconic for her unique style and openness about her sexuality – before leaving Berlin, she had enjoyed the drag ball scene of the 1920s and visiting gay bars. She defied gender norms with her love of men's suits, while also occasionally taking on a more feminine appearance. It's quite possible that, if queer language and identities had been a little more prominent, Dietrich may have identified as gender non-binary or non-conforming. Today, Dietrich may also have identified as polyamorous, with her many affairs no secret from her husband, Rudolf Sieber. Dietrich even made a habit of showing letters from her lovers to her husband. Her affairs would also commonly overlap with one another. Dietrich bore no shame in an era where polyamory was not commonplace and she could perhaps be recognized for normalizing it. She was known to pursue women with more passion than she did men, making no secret of her bisexuality.

Dietrich passed away in 1992, leaving behind the legacy of a sex-positive queer role model.

"THERE IS A GIGANTIC DIFFERENCE BETWEEN EARNING A GREAT DEAL OF MONEY AND BEING RICH."

THEIR AWESOME ACHIEVEMENTS

→ Saved the lives of many German and French exiles by housing them during World War Two.

→ Honoured with a star on the Hollywood Walk of Fame in 1960.

→ Received the Special David accolade at the David di Donatello Awards for her performance in the film *Judgement at Nuremberg* in 1962.

→ Received the Honorary Award at the German Film Awards in 1980.

→ Pursued many lovers of different genders, without ever fearing judgement for her choices. Though she never specifically advocated for LGBTQ issues, she certainly did a lot for bisexual visibility.

→ Made no secret of her affairs and would likely have identified as polyamorous.

"I DRESS FOR THE IMAGE. NOT FOR MYSELF, NOT FOR THE PUBLIC, NOT FOR FASHION, NOT FOR MEN."

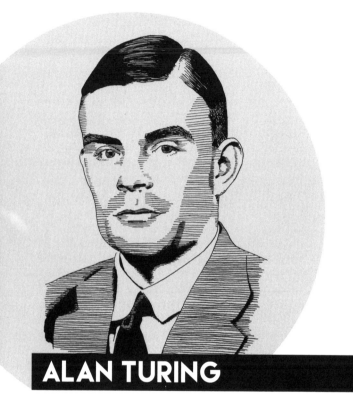

ALAN TURING

1912–54

SUPERPOWERS

Codebreaker, mathematician, computer scientist.

THEIR INCREDIBLE STORY

Codebreaker and mathematician Alan Turing is remembered for his efforts during World War Two, for his proficiency in mathematics and the advances he made in computer science, including the "Turing test" for computer intelligence that is still used today. Sadly, he is also remembered for his conviction as a homosexual and his subsequent treatment. He left behind a legacy that would eventually see a posthumous pardon bestowed upon all men convicted of homosexual acts in the UK.

Turing studied as an undergraduate at King's College, Cambridge, graduating in 1934, and would later become involved with the University of Manchester's Computing Machine Laboratory. During World War Two, Turing worked as a codebreaker as part of the Government Code and Cypher School (now known as GCHQ). He developed techniques to break German ciphers and provided invaluable intelligence, with groundwork laid by Polish codebreakers Jerzy Różycki, Henryk Zygalski and Marian Rejewski; while the British were still trying to break the codes using linguistics, these Polish codebreakers realized it was imperative to use mathematics to decipher the code patterns. Utilizing the information provided by the codebreakers, Turing's work ultimately helped win the war, helping the Allied forces in several crucial engagements. It's estimated that Turing's efforts shorted the war in

Europe by approximately two years and saved more than 14 million lives.

Sadly, despite Turing's war efforts, his relationship with Arnold Murray was discovered when police came to Turing's home following a reported burglary. Both men were convicted of homosexual acts in 1952. Turing pled guilty under advisement, after he was presented with the choice of imprisonment or probation on the condition of chemical castration. He chose the latter, despite the fact the hormone treatment would have drastic effects on his body. Due to the conviction, Turing had his security clearance revoked, was unable to continue his work with the government and was prohibited from discussing his previous work.

In 1954, two years after his conviction, Turing was found dead. Though the circumstances of his death have long been questioned, it is believed he killed himself. In 2013, he was posthumously pardoned of gross indecency, following a campaign by MP John Leech who declared it "utterly disgusting and ultimately just embarrassing" that Turing's conviction had been upheld for so long in spite of his war efforts. Leech continued his campaign after Turing's pardon, seeking a general pardon for all men convicted of homosexuality, and he succeeded – in 2017, approximately 50,000 men convicted of homosexual acts were posthumously pardoned under the Alan Turing Law, an informal term for a clause contained within the Policing and Crime Act of 2017.

THEIR AWESOME ACHIEVEMENTS

➜ Developed techniques in computer science that are still used today, such as the Turing test.

➜ Developed codebreaking techniques that would ultimately help win the war by deciphering German ciphers, providing invaluable intelligence to the allied forces. His contributions shortened the war in Europe by years and saved a drastic number of lives as a result.

➜ Honoured with a number of concepts, institutions and lectures named after him, such as the Turing test, the Turing Institute and the Turing degree.

➜ Posthumously pardoned along with other men convicted of homosexuality, under the Policing and Crime Act 2017, following a specific clause known as the Alan Turing law.

"THOSE WHO CAN IMAGINE ANYTHING, CAN CREATE THE IMPOSSIBLE."

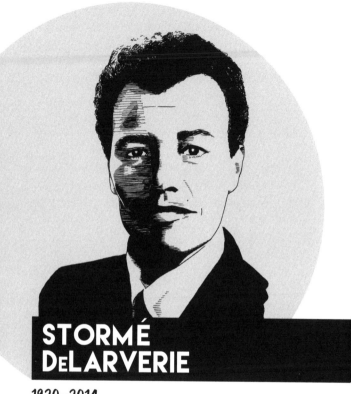

STORMÉ DeLARVERIE

1920–2014

SUPERPOWERS

Guardian of lesbians, singer, drag king, Stonewall participant.

THEIR INCREDIBLE STORY

Known as the "guardian of the lesbians" for her work in later life protecting fellow queer women, Stormé DeLarverie was one of the key figures in the Stonewall uprising, and one of the many queer women of colour we now have to thank for the queer civil rights movement that followed. DeLarverie was a butch lesbian and performed as a drag king before going on to become a bouncer at various New York bars.

DeLarverie had a difficult upbringing, being both queer and of mixed racial heritage. She was abused by her peers because of her parents' interracial relationship, leading her father to enrol her in private schooling for her protection. She later worked as a performer and drag king; she had been warned that drag would ruin her career as a singer, but she retained a regular performance spot at the Jewel Box in Miami for 14 years.

Most stories of the Stonewall uprising rely on eye-witness accounts, so there are inevitably some inconsistencies, but it is clear that DeLarverie was heavily involved in the events that sparked the uprising. The story goes, as told by witnesses and DeLarverie herself, that she was handcuffed during a police raid of the Stonewall Inn in Greenwich Village, New York City, and roughly escorted out. She managed to escape back into the bar several times, rallying the crowd. Witnesses saw the rough treatment of DeLarverie, who had been hit on the head for claiming her cuffs were too tight, and the crowd stepped in to help her and fight back.

Not long after the Stonewall uprising, DeLarverie's partner Diana, a dancer, passed away. DeLarverie almost completely stopped performing at this point, carrying a photo of Diana with her at all times.

She dedicated most of the rest of her life to the protection of other queer people, particularly women, from the abuse she had endured. She worked as a bouncer at several lesbian bars in New York, and volunteered as a street patroller – "the guardian of the lesbians in the Village". During DeLarverie's street patrols she usually carried a baseball bat and looked out for any signs of bullying and abuse – what she called "ugliness" – directed at the queer community (particularly lesbians). DeLarverie would also ensure the safety of others at Pride parades, and would often hold benefits for abused women and children. Close friend Lisa Cannistraci said that DeLarverie kept up her security operations until she was 85 years old and some even referred to her as a "gay superhero" for her protective actions.

In 2014, DeLarverie died in a nursing home. Despite suffering from dementia, memories of her childhood and the Stonewall uprising never dimmed.

THEIR AWESOME ACHIEVEMENTS

→ Played a key role in the Stonewall uprising, encouraging the community to take action against the police mistreatment of LGBTQ people.

→ Made clear that Stonewall was an uprising and a revolution, and that "riot" was a name given to the event in negativity.

→ Was a successful drag king act for 14 years despite claims it would end her career.

→ Became a protector of the LGBTQ community, particularly women and young people, and remained so until she was in her eighties.

"I CAN SPOT UGLY IN A MINUTE. NO PEOPLE EVEN PULL IT AROUND ME THAT KNOW ME. THEY'LL JUST WALK AWAY, AND THAT'S A GOOD THING TO DO BECAUSE I'LL EITHER PICK UP THE PHONE OR I'LL NAIL YOU."

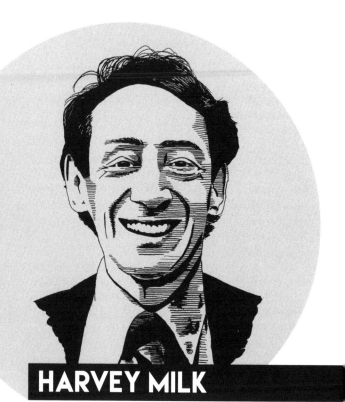

HARVEY MILK

1930–78

SUPERPOWERS

Queer politician, LGBTQ rights activist, uniter of queer voices.

THEIR INCREDIBLE STORY

Harvey Milk was the first openly gay elected official in California and an instrumental figure in LGBTQ rights in the USA. Though Milk's LGBTQ activism didn't come until later in his political career, he had a huge impact in a short time.

Milk's political career in San Francisco had a rocky start, but he soon became the self-styled Mayor of Castro Street by allying himself with organized labour unions and used that relationship to provide more work opportunities for gay residents. Along with other gay business owners in the area, he formed the Castro Village Association, encouraging queer businesses to work together.

Shortly afterward, Milk was appointed to the Board of Permit Appeals in San Francisco by Mayor George Moscone, becoming the first openly gay commissioner in US history. However, before long, Milk decided to run for California State Assembly and Moscone was forced to fire him, as neither elected nor appointed officials were allowed to run campaigns while performing their duties.

When Milk failed in his bid for State Assembly and sensed that he wouldn't gain support from the existing LGBT Democratic Club, he formed the Harvey Milk LGBT Democratic Club. One of the club's first campaigns took the form of a demonstration at a speech by Vice President of the USA Walter Mondale, urging Mondale to speak on gay rights. Though Mondale did not acquiesce, the new LGBT Democratic Club had proven itself to have a strong voice.

Milk's final campaign in 1977 saw him elected to the San Francisco Board of Supervisors. However, his openness in supporting queer rights throughout the campaign drew a lot of negative attention including violent death threats. Milk even recorded a message to leave behind in the event of his assassination, saying, "If a bullet should enter my brain, let that bullet destroy every closet door."

Milk's visibility also brought some other resistance – from the people pushing California Proposition 6 – a law that would ban LGBTQ people from working in public schools. Milk urged queer people nationwide to come out and be visible, believing that if they were open to their friends, family and colleagues, people would see the damaging effects Proposition 6 would have on their queer loved ones. Proposition 6 was defeated in 1978.

Tragically, in 1978, Harvey Milk was assassinated, along with Mayor Moscone, by a member of the Board of Supervisors, Dan White. White and Milk had frequently clashed on city issues.

Harvey Milk had a profound impact on LGBTQ and progressive politics. He left behind a legacy that raised the visibility of queer people and gave them a voice to speak in unison.

THEIR AWESOME ACHIEVEMENTS

→ First openly gay elected official in California.

→ Organized the gay bars of Castro Street to participate in union strikes against breweries that refused to sign union contracts (Coors in particular).

→ Founded the Castro Village Association to support queer businesses and to encourage the employment of more gay men.

→ Introduced the Gay Rights Law to prohibit discrimination in housing and employment.

→ Drove thousands to register to vote.

→ Prevented Proposition 6 from entering into California law, which would have prevented LGBTQ people working in public schools.

"BUT ONCE AND FOR ALL, BREAK DOWN THE MYTHS. DESTROY THE LIES AND DISTORTIONS. FOR YOUR SAKE. FOR THEIR SAKE."

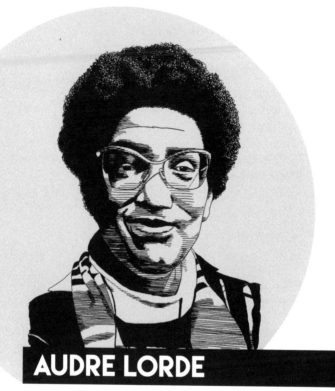

AUDRE LORDE

1934–92

SUPERPOWERS

Civil rights activist, feminist, introducer of intersectionality in feminism, poet, lesbian, mother.

THEIR INCREDIBLE STORY

Despite being declared legally blind due to her near-sightedness, Audre Lorde learned how to read and write at an early age. She wrote poetry from a young age and continued to do so throughout her life. She wrote her first poems at high school and participated in workshops organized by the Harlem Writers' Guild, which recognized those who felt excluded from the mainstream literary culture of New York due to their African-American heritage.

Lorde became estranged from her family after graduation, moved to Connecticut and began to explore her sexual identity. She spent a year studying at the National University of Mexico in 1954, where she claimed to have grown as both a poet and a lesbian, and upon her return to New York, became involved with the gay culture in Greenwich Village. Although Lorde self-identified as a lesbian, she did briefly marry attorney Edwin Rollins in 1962. Their marriage was unconventional, particularly for the time, due to being an interracial marriage, and they had two children, Elizabeth and Jonathan. A few years into their marriage, Lorde began a teaching career at Tougaloo College in Mississippi, inspiring a new generation of black poets. It was here that she fell in love with a woman – Frances Clayton. This led to Lorde and Rollins' divorce in 1970 and Lorde building a family life with Clayton, Elizabeth and Jonathan.

Lorde was active in the civil rights, pacifist and feminist movements, and her poetry reflected all of these identities and struggles. In her essays, most notably in *Age, Race, Class and Sex: Women Redefining Difference*, Lorde focused on the many layers that make up the overall identity and experience of an individual – race, age, gender, sexuality and even health – and the importance of the oppressed teaching the oppressor their mistakes. This was something that Lorde was determined to do in regard to white-focused feminism. This introduced the idea of intersectionality to feminism, with several identities each factoring into the individual's lived experience. Later, intersectionality would also introduce transgender identities. To that end, Lorde was critical of the feminist movement in the 1960s and took particular issue with the racism of feminists only focusing on the issues faced by middle-class white women. Lorde's theories were unpopular and she bore the brunt of anger from the existing feminist movement. Today, however, intersectionality is a crucial part of feminism.

Lorde identified in her own words as "black, lesbian, mother, poet", refusing to let her identity be put into one box. In 1992, after a 14-year battle with cancer, a fight that Lorde wrote much about, she died. Though her theories on intersectional feminism were unpopular in her lifetime, the impact of her theories is at last being recognized and respected today.

THEIR AWESOME ACHIEVEMENTS

➜ Introduced intersectional philosophy to feminism; the idea that as well as gender, race, class, sexuality and many other factors impact someone's experience as a woman.

➜ Changed the understanding of identity – that no person could be put into one box and instead the self was made up of several different identities.

➜ Wrote many inspiring poems, journals and theories despite having been declared legally blind.

➜ Won the American Library Association's Gay Caucus Book of the Year award for *The Cancer Journals* in 1981, and the American Book Award for *A Burst of Light* in 1989. Became the Poet Laureate of New York in 1991 and received the Publishing Triangle Bill Whitehead Award for Lifetime Achievement in 1992.

➜ The Publishing Triangle Audre Lorde Award for works of lesbian poetry was created in her honour in 2001.

"IT IS NOT OUR DIFFERENCES THAT DIVIDE US. IT IS OUR INABILITY TO RECOGNIZE, ACCEPT AND CELEBRATE THOSE DIFFERENCES."

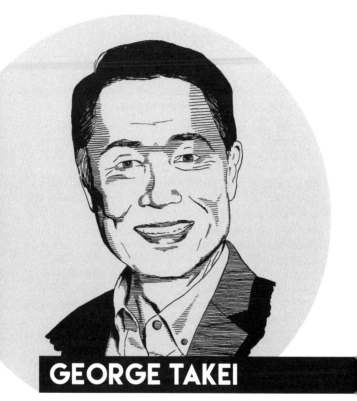

GEORGE TAKEI

1937–PRESENT

SUPERPOWERS

Internment camp survivor, iconic actor, equal marriage advocate.

THEIR INCREDIBLE STORY

Many know him as Lt Hikaru Sulu from *Star Trek*, others know him as an LGBTQ icon. George Takei is well remembered for his public coming out and for two simple words: "oh my."

Along with many Japanese Americans of his generation, following the Japanese bombing of Pearl Harbour, Takei and his family were placed in an internment camp. They remained in the camp for three years and were released when he was eight years old.

When the war ended, Takei and his family returned to Los Angeles. After graduating with a Masters in theatre, he took on small roles in Hollywood, before landing a leading role in an episode of *The Twilight Zone* in 1964. One year later, he landed his standout role as Sulu in *Star Trek*. He also went on to play Sulu in *Star Trek: The Animated Series* and the first six *Star Trek* films.

For the majority of his acting career, Takei hid his sexuality. He had heard the story of once-prominent actor Tab Hunter being outed as gay and then disappearing from the Hollywood scene. It was incredibly difficult for Takei to hide that part of who he was for so long – he would go to gay bars where he could be himself, although in the time before the Stonewall uprising he felt that being at the mercy of the police in public was not dissimilar to being in the internment camp.

Coming out publicly in 2005 was an act of protest for Takei, when Arnold Schwarzenegger, then governor of California, vetoed a same-sex marriage bill and blocked progress for the LGBTQ community of California. Takei felt particularly angry as Schwarzenegger had shown allegiance to the LGBTQ community throughout his campaign. The community felt that Schwarzenegger had betrayed them. Same-sex marriage was not legalized in California until 2013.

Takei had worried that coming out as gay would end his career, however, since then his career has truly blossomed. Takei is still welcomed with open arms at *Star Trek* conventions, signing hundreds of autographs for his adoring fans. In 2014 he took part in filming the documentary *To Be Takei* (cleverly pointing out the pun with the tag line, "It's okay to be Takei"). The documentary explores the history of his career in film and television, including his struggles with coming out and his life with his husband Brad Takei. He still speaks out for LGBTQ rights and continues to enjoy being his unapologetic queer self.

"GAYS AND LESBIANS HAVE BEEN STEREOTYPED BY SOCIETY. BY SHARING OUR EXPERIENCES – BOTH GOOD AND BAD, ENRICHING AND UNHAPPY – WE HUMANIZE WHO WE ARE."

THEIR AWESOME ACHIEVEMENTS

→ Honoured with a star on the Hollywood Walk of Fame in 1986.

→ Issued an Order of the Rising Sun, Gold Rays with Rosette by the Japanese government for his contributions to US–Japanese relations. Also received the Distinguished Medal of Honour for Lifetime Achievement and Public Service from the Japanese American National Museum in 2015.

→ Won many awards for his portrayal of Japanese characters in cinema and his LGBTQ advocacy, including a Lifetime Achievement Award from the San Diego Asian Film Festival in 2007, the LGBT Humanist Award from the American Humanist Association in 2012 and the Vito Russo Award from GLAAD for promoting LGBTQ equality in 2014.

→ Awarded an Honorary Doctorate of Humane Letters from California State University.

→ Bravely came out publicly, after a lifetime of worrying for both his safety and career due to his sexuality.

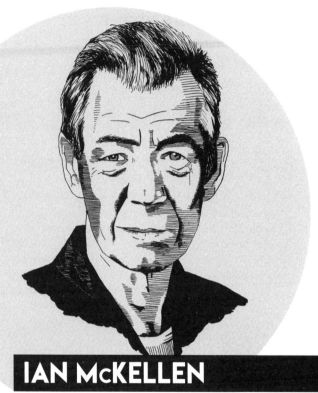

IAN McKELLEN

1939–PRESENT

SUPERPOWERS

Queer wizard, LGBTQ rights activist, Stonewall founder.

THEIR INCREDIBLE STORY

The gay wizard himself, Sir Ian McKellen is widely recognized for his role as Gandalf in Peter Jackson's film adaptations of *The Lord of the Rings*. However, McKellen is a person of many achievements beyond acting – he is also a prominent LGBTQ rights activist.

In 1988, McKellen came out publicly during a BBC Radio 3 discussion centred on the controversial Section 28 of the Local Government Act 1988. Section 28 was a clause that would forbid the "promotion" of homosexuality in Britain in any published material, with a particular focus on ensuring homosexuality wasn't taught about in schools. The clause referred to homosexuality as a "pretended family relationship".

McKellen's coming out was both an act of bravery and defiance. As the clause prevented the promotion of homosexuality, by coming out publicly McKellen was breaking that law. When asked if he would like to see Section 28 abolished, McKellen replied: "I certainly would. It's offensive to anyone who is, like myself, homosexual, apart from the whole business of what can and cannot be taught to children."

McKellen has expressed regret in not coming out sooner, wishing he had been more involved with LGBTQ rights earlier on. However, he hit the ground running in the fight; almost immediately afterward, he visited the UK environment secretary at the time, Michael Howard, to lobby against Section 28.

Howard's position remained unchanged, though he still asked McKellen for an autograph for his children. McKellen signed the autograph, "Fuck off – I'm gay."

McKellen co-founded Stonewall in 1989, the UK LGBTQ charity that takes its name from the Stonewall uprising in New York City in 1969. The charity, whose current motto is "acceptance without exception", continues to fight for the rights of LGBTQ individuals. Its first successful campaign was to lift the ban of LGBTQ people serving in the armed forces, something that was achieved in 1999.

No stranger to the Pride movement, McKellen is a patron of Pride London and Oxford Pride, and has been grand marshal of the Pride marches in Manchester and San Francisco. He is also a patron of the LGBT Foundation charity, and the Friends and Families of Lesbians and Gays (FFLAG) organization, appearing in their *Parents Talking* video.

Despite an impressive acting career, McKellen has said he wants to be remembered for his LGBTQ rights activism. In an interview with *Pink News* in 2017, he said: "I'm very proud of my small contributions in changing the law in this country and changing the attitudes, all for the better. And I suppose in the scheme of things that is more important and the more merit and longer lasting than any acting I have ever done."

THEIR AWESOME ACHIEVEMENTS

➔ Received a knighthood in 1991.

➔ Founded the Stonewall charity.

➔ Spoke out and campaigned against the damaging Section 28 clause in British law.

➔ Campaigned with Stonewall – and succeeded – to lift the ban on LGBTQ people serving in the British Armed Forces.

➔ Received the Pride International Film Festival Lifetime Achievement and Distinction Award.

➔ Won two Screen Actors Guild awards for *The Lord of the Rings: The Fellowship of the Ring* and a Golden Globe for *Rasputin: Dark Servant of Destiny.*

➔ Won six Oliver Awards for his theatre performances.

"IT WAS WRONGLY ASSUMED THAT I WISHED TO BECOME SOME SORT OF LEADER AMONG GAY ACTIVISTS, WHEREAS IN REALITY I WAS HAPPIER TO BE A FOOT SOLDIER."

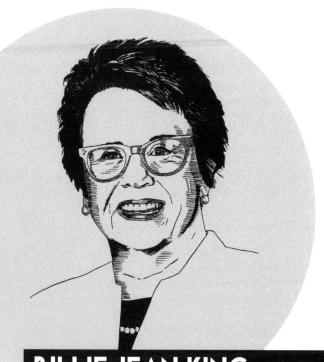

BILLIE JEAN KING

1943–PRESENT

SUPERPOWERS

Battle of the Sexes winner, feminist, tennis reformer.

THEIR INCREDIBLE STORY

Billie Jean King is one of tennis's feminist icons – and not just for winning the infamous Battle of the Sexes. Throughout her career she focused on gender equality and smashing the glass ceiling of the tennis world.

King's battle for equality within tennis began when she was only 12. She noticed the abundance of white on the playing field, from the clothing and equipment to the competitors. She realized this had to change – for everyone – and would spend her career accomplishing this goal.

In 1973, at the age of 29, King won the famous Battle of the Sexes against retired former men's tennis champion Bobby Riggs, who had baited her by claiming that female players were inferior and that a woman would not be able to beat him. King initially refused to accept the challenge, but reconsidered when Riggs won against Margaret Court who at the time was the top female tennis player in the world. King proved, as she had in her career up until then, that women were not to be underestimated on the court.

In 1970, along with eight other women tennis players, King formed the "Original 9" and fought for equal pay in tennis regardless of gender. Along with the Original 9, King founded the Virginia Slims Circuit – the first professional women's tennis tour – and in 1973, she became the president of the

Women's Tennis Association. King's actions opened the sport up to people of all backgrounds and made the playing field much more open, even for women – not just rich white men.

King fought to take tennis to a new level of professionalism, and fought to demolish the shady deals in which big-name players were paid to ensure they would enter the existing tournaments and which paid male players drastically more than women (despite winning the respective singles titles in the 1972 US Open, King earned $15,000 less than Ilie Năstase). Deciding she wouldn't let this slide, King announced that she would not enter the tournament the following year unless men and women players were paid equally, and in 1973, the US Open became the first tournament to do this.

During the 1970s, King began a secret relationship with Marilyn Barnett. Their relationship was troublesome and in 1979 they separated. In 1981 King was publicly outed when Barnett took legal action against her that exposed details of their relationship. King said the incident was horrible and that she wasn't ready to be publicly out, though she did not want to deny or hide her identity. King claimed it took "tons of therapy" for her to finally become comfortable with her sexuality at the age of 51. Reflecting on the incident, King insisted that no one should out anyone and that people should only come out when they are ready.

King has said that in today's more progressive times, coming out would have been much easier. She has expressed much respect for the millennial generation, realizing they are largely to thank for today's inclusivity. But King herself was responsible for the first steps that took tennis as a profession to a much more inclusive place.

THEIR AWESOME ACHIEVEMENTS

→ Won the Battle of the Sexes match in 1973 and put women on the map in tennis.

→ Campaigned tirelessly for tennis to be a more inclusive and professional sport.

→ Highlighted the gender pay inequality of the sport, which would inspire similar investigations in other fields.

→ Awarded Female Athlete of the Year by the Associated Press in 1967 and 1973, Sportsperson of the Year by *Sports Illustrated* in 1972 and inducted into the International Tennis Hall of Fame in 1987.

→ Honoured with the Arthur Ashe Courage Award in 1999, inducted into the National Gay and Lesbian Sports Hall of Fame in 2000, and awarded the *Glamour* Lifetime Achievement Award in 2006 and the Presidential Medal of Freedom in 2009.

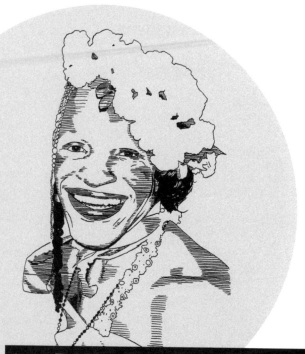

MARSHA P. JOHNSON

1945–92

SUPERPOWERS

Stonewall uprising instigator, co-founder of STAR,
gender non-conformer, queer liberation activist.

THEIR INCREDIBLE STORY

Without Marsha P. Johnson – the activist most commonly remembered for her role in the Stonewall uprising – and other founding members of the Gay Liberation Front, the Pride movement of today may not exist.

Johnson grew up in a family largely unaware of the LGBTQ community, except for her mother's view that being gay was "lower than a dog". After graduating from Edison High School, Johnson left for New York City, where she became involved in the drag scene. When talking about her drag style, Johnson said she didn't consider it to be serious or "high drag" as she couldn't afford expensive clothing, accessories or make-up. Her identity was variable: she would identify as gay, a transvestite and a queen, and she described her drag as gender non-conforming. Johnson used female pronouns but didn't discuss her gender identity at length. Many historians and academics studying queer history theorize that had the language been more widely used, she would have identified as transgender.

When the Stonewall Inn began to allow women and drag queens into the venue, Johnson was one of the first drag queens to frequent the bar. As with many gay bars in the 1960s, the Stonewall was subject to police raids due to the legal restrictions on homosexuality at the time. In 1969 Johnson arrived at the bar in the early hours of the morning to find the resistance had already begun, and the Stonewall uprising had been started by Stormé DeLarverie earlier that night (see page 23). Johnson joined in with the resistance efforts, screaming, "I got my civil rights!", climbing a lamppost and dropping a brick on a police car in protest.

The uprising led to demonstrations in Greenwich Village, which saw between 500 and 1,000 protesters gather outside the Stonewall Inn. After the uprising, Johnson co-founded the Gay Liberation Front and took part in one of the first Pride rallies in 1970. Johnson co-founded the Street Transvestite Action Revolutionaries (STAR) organization – which offered shelter to the LGBTQ homeless youth of New York, California, Chicago and England – along with Sylvia Rivera. Together, Johnson and Rivera became well-known figures in the LGBTQ community of New York and at the early Pride rallies.

In 1992, Johnson was found dead in the Hudson River. Her death was ruled a suicide by police, despite a suspicious-looking head wound and claims that she wasn't suicidal. After much campaigning by LGBTQ rights activist Mariah Cruz, in 2012, the Johnson's case was successfully reopened as a potential homicide.

It's important to remember Johnson's work in a world that continues to erase transgender experiences, particularly those of people of colour. Johnson fought proudly for the rights of the whole

LGBTQ community as a prominent figure in the Gay Liberation Front, and to this day, her bravery in the Stonewall uprising still inspires LGBTQ rights activists around the world.

THEIR AWESOME ACHIEVEMENTS

→ Stood up for the civil rights of the LGBTQ community at the Stonewall uprising.

→ Kick-started a revolution that saw LGBTQ rights recognized by the wider community.

→ Co-founded the STAR organization, which assisted homeless LGBTQ people in cities across the US and England.

→ Still inspires the fight for LGBTQ civil rights worldwide and is still fondly remembered at Pride marches that came about as a result of the events at Stonewall.

"WHAT'S THE POINT OF COMPLAINING? IT DON'T GET YOU NOWHERE."

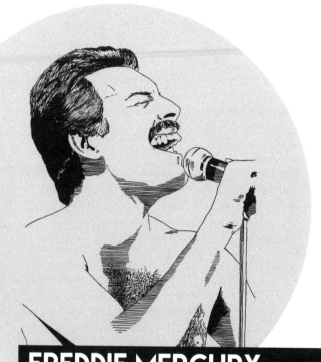

FREDDIE MERCURY

1946–91

THEIR SUPERPOWERS

Unapologetically and visibly queer songwriter, greatest singer in the history of pop music.

THEIR INCREDIBLE STORY

Freddie Mercury was the unapologetically flamboyant lead vocalist of British rock band, Queen; the person who bestowed upon us classic hits like "Killer Queen", an impressive four-octave vocal range and some iconic looks to boot.

Having admired the stylings of Brian May and Roger Taylor in their band Smile, Mercury encouraged the pair to become more experimental and join him – and thus, Queen was born in 1970. (Bassist John Deacon completed what would be the long-time Queen line-up in 1971.) Queen produced some of the most well-remembered rock hits of the era, such as "Bohemian Rhapsody" and "I Want to Break Free". Mercury's performance with Queen at Live Aid 1985 is widely remembered as one of his most impressive, in which he commanded the undivided attention of the huge audience. A note sustained by Mercury during an a capella segment of this performance would be remembered as "the note heard around the world".

Although Mercury's friends knew him to be shyer than his on-stage persona suggested, he was also known to enjoy a party. Though he attended many, one of his most notable nights involved helping Princess Diana dodge the tabloid photographers to attend a party at the then infamous gay bar, the Royal Vauxhall Tavern. Mercury, actress Cleo Rocos and Kenny Everett disguised the princess as a gay male model to smuggle her in. The disguise worked, partially due to Mercury's distracting star power.

Mercury's sexuality has often been a topic of debate. Tabloid journalists would constantly attempt to out him, but he saw no need to explain his lifestyle. This made Mercury something of an LGBTQ inspiration, never hiding his authentic self and refusing to justify his sexuality. This was during a time when homosexuality had only recently been decriminalized, with the LGBTQ community often still treated with contempt. Mercury showed the world that being queer wasn't something to be ashamed of.

Freddie Mercury's tragic and untimely death in 1991 from AIDS represented an important event in the history of the disease, due to Mercury's high profile. The remaining members of Queen founded the Mercury Phoenix Trust in his memory and since then have raised millions for various AIDS charities. Having been a close friend of Mercury's until his death, Princess Diana became a patron for the National AIDS Trust and devoted her efforts to promoting awareness of HIV. The day before his death, Mercury said he hoped that people worldwide would join him in the fight against the disease.

"I WON'T BE A ROCK STAR. I WILL BE A LEGEND."

THEIR AWESOME ACHIEVEMENTS

➔ Wrote many of Queen's greatest hits, to roaring success, including "I Want to Break Free", "Bohemian Rhapsody", "Crazy Little Thing Called Love" and more.

➔ Won many awards as frontman of Queen, including the Brit Awards Best British Single for "Bohemian Rhapsody" in 1977 and Outstanding Contribution to Music in 1990.

➔ Performed to one of the largest audiences – and the largest TV audience at the time – at Live Aid in 1985, simultaneously bringing Queen back into the spotlight.

➔ Performed live at an estimated 700 concerts throughout his career.

➔ Ultimately raised awareness of HIV and AIDS with his dying wish: "I hope everyone will join with me, my doctors and all those worldwide in the fight against this terrible disease."

➔ Posthumously awarded Brit Award for Outstanding Contribution to Music in 1992.

"I ALWAYS KNEW I WAS A STAR. AND NOW, THE REST OF THE WORLD SEEMS TO AGREE WITH ME."

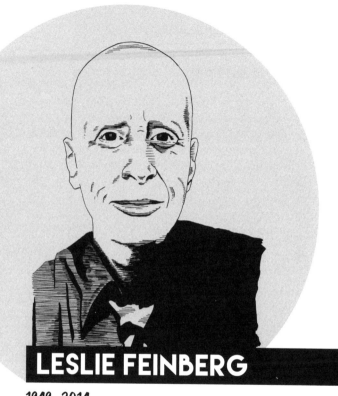

LESLIE FEINBERG

1949–2014

SUPERPOWERS

Transgender language pioneer, gender non-conformer, writer.

THEIR INCREDIBLE STORY

Leslie Feinberg was a gender non-conforming author and transgender rights activist. Feinberg identified with gender-inclusive pronouns, zie and hir. Hir work as an author had a huge impact on the understanding of transgender experiences with hir first novel, *Stone Butch Blues*, considered to be particularly groundbreaking in this regard. Hir words helped open readers' eyes and minds to queer identities, and offered transgender and gender non-conforming readers an experience more relatable than any they had come across before.

Feinberg grew up in Buffalo, New York. Zie began supporting hirself at a young age, working while in high school. Eventually zie stopped attending classes, though zie still received hir diploma. When Feinberg started to frequent the gay bars of Buffalo, hir family became hostile due to hir gender presentation and sexuality. Zie moved away from hir family and would later legally disown them. Feinberg experienced many difficulties due to hir gender identity and expression, including finding stable employment, and zie had to rely on various odd jobs to get by.

Though Feinberg was not involved in the Stonewall uprising, zie expressed regret at missing the events, saying, "I was mad I missed it, I was ready to fight." Feinberg's experiences at the hands of the police in

Buffalo were not dissimilar to those at Stonewall, so zie was just as angry as those taking part.

These experiences went on to shape Feinberg's career as an author and zie wrote *Stone Butch Blues*, published in 1993, as a result. Feinberg was always clear that the book was not autobiographical and on the 20th anniversary of its publication, called it "a work of fiction, written by an author who has lived the non-fiction".

As a work of fiction, *Stone Butch Blues* is considered to be one of the most important and accurate works to relate transgender experiences, and in reaching a wide audience it increased both visibility and understanding of transgender lives.

Feinberg's non-fiction writings were equally important, helping to define language surrounding transgender identities. Zie would define "transgender" as "all people who cross the cultural boundaries of gender", while also describing transgender people as an oppressed group in need of civil rights advancement.

In later life, Feinberg experienced medical discrimination due to hir gender identity, almost dying on one occasion. Zie remained a protestor for transgender rights until hir death in 2014. Feinberg gave language to the transgender experience that previously hadn't existed and shared aspects of hir journey to validate transgender lives.

THEIR AWESOME ACHIEVEMENTS

→ Won the American Library Association Gay, Lesbian and Bisexual Book Award for *Stone Butch Blues* in 1994.

→ Changed and developed the language of transgender experience.

→ Redefined and developed understanding of transgender individuals.

→ Inspired a generation of transgender, gender queer and gender non-binary people to find strength and beauty within themselves.

→ Inspired a generation of activists for LGBTQ causes.

"I CARE WHICH PRONOUN IS USED, BUT PEOPLE HAVE BEEN RESPECTFUL TO ME WITH THE WRONG PRONOUN AND DISRESPECTFUL WITH THE RIGHT ONE. IT MATTERS WHETHER SOMEONE IS USING THE PRONOUN AS A BIGOT, OR IF THEY ARE TRYING TO DEMONSTRATE RESPECT."

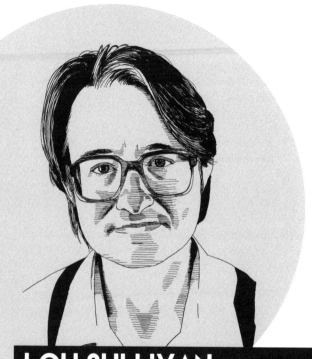

LOU SULLIVAN

1951–91

SUPERPOWERS

FTM pioneer, transgender male rights activist, gender and sexuality separatist.

THEIR INCREDIBLE STORY

Author and transgender activist Lou Sullivan is largely recognized for his work in distinguishing gender identity and sexuality as separate concepts. He pioneered the female-to-male (FTM) transgender movement of the 1980s and worked closely with the transgender male community to ensure they had the support they needed during their transitions.

Transgender rights activism had largely focused on the male-to-female (MTF) transgender community, so Sullivan focused his efforts on supporting those transitioning FTM. Sullivan provided peer counselling through the Janus Information Facility of San Francisco, an organization that provided support to the transgender community. Sullivan also wrote the first ever guidebook for FTM individuals, providing important information that had been previously unavailable. To further provide understanding of FTM experiences, Sullivan penned the biography of a prominent FTM figure in San Francisco – *From Female to Male: The Life of Jack Bee Garland.*

As a gay transgender man, Sullivan worked hard to raise awareness of transgender individuals who identified as homosexual. Many did not recognize that gender identity and sexuality were separate, believing in the heteronormative ideal that men were attracted to women and vice versa, so if a person's gender identity were to change their sexuality would change accordingly. Sullivan challenged this idea, and spent a lifetime defining sexuality and gender identity as separate concepts.

Sullivan fought for the American Psychiatric Association and the World Professional Association for Transgender Health to recognize his identity as a gay transgender man. He campaigned for sexual orientation to be removed from the criteria when diagnosing gender identity disorder, so fewer barricades would be presented for FTM individuals seeking hormone treatments and surgery.

Sullivan wrote about these issues as part of the Golden Gate Girls/Guys organization (later renamed the Gateway Gender Alliance), serving as the editor of the newsletter in 1979. The organization went on to be one of the first to support FTM individuals thanks to Sullivan's involvement. Sullivan was also a founder of the GLBT Historical Society where many of his papers are often displayed in exhibitions.

In 1986 Sullivan was diagnosed with HIV and given just one year to live. He lived for another five years and died in 1991. Sullivan said at the time: "I took a certain pleasure in informing the gender clinic that even though their programme told me I could not live as a gay man, it looks like I'm going to die like one." His diagnosis supported his identity to those who denied it.

THEIR AWESOME ACHIEVEMENTS

➜ Provided research and education to the FTM community that had previously been non-existent.

➜ Supported and made visible the FTM community at a time when most transgender research and education concerned MTF individuals.

➜ Wrote the first guidebook for FTM individuals.

➜ Campaigned to remove sexual orientation from the criteria when diagnosing gender identity disorder.

➜ Made people aware that gender identity and sexual orientation are two exclusive concepts and do not impact one another.

➜ Founded the GLBT Historical Society.

"HOW STRANGE IT SEEMS THAT EDUCATION, IN PRACTICE, SO OFTEN MEANS SUPPRESSION: THAT INSTEAD OF LEADING THE MIND OUTWARD TO THE LIGHT OF DAY IT CROWDS THINGS IN UPON IT THAT DARKEN AND WEARY IT."

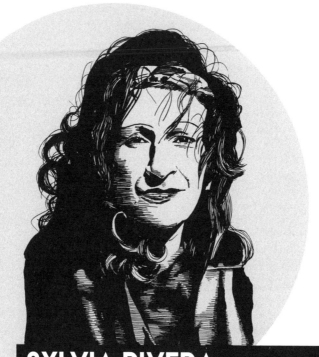

SYLVIA RIVERA

1951–2002

SUPERPOWERS

Stonewall instigator, LGBTQ and trans rights pioneer, queer visibility advocate.

THEIR INCREDIBLE STORY

Rivera was a gender-fluid drag queen who was heavily involved in the Stonewall uprising along with Marsha P. Johnson (see page 46), with both reported to have resisted during a police raid on the Stonewall Inn in 1969. Following the uprising, the pair formed Street Transvestite Action Revolutionaries (STAR), which provided assistance to LGBTQ homeless youth, and focused on helping drag queens and people of colour. Together they opened STAR House, a shelter for homeless transgender youth, queens and hustlers.

Rivera became one of America's first transgender rights activists, working tirelessly for civil rights and justice for the LGBTQ community, particularly for minority queer identities. She fought for and successfully achieved the Sexual Orientation Non-Discrimination Act of New York in 1971 – a great victory for the LGBTQ community as businesses, employers and educators could no longer discriminate on the basis of someone's sexuality. This meant there were fewer barriers for queer people seeking housing.

Rivera was also heavily involved in the campaign for the New York City Gay Rights Bill, insisting that drag queens and gender non-conforming people be included within the legislation. Rivera even went to the length of scaling the walls of City Hall in full make-up, a dress and heels, to crash a meeting about the proposal. Her famous words, "Hell hath no fury like a drag queen scorned," came in response to learning that the bill had not included the language that would protect those gender non-conformists she had fought for.

In spite of her activism, Rivera was not fully accepted by the mainstream gay civil rights movement – she wasn't white, she wasn't cisgender (someone who identifies as the gender they were assigned at birth) and she certainly wasn't quiet and ready to assimilate. While making her way to the stage at the fourth annual Christopher Street Liberation Day Rally in 1973, she was blocked and physically attacked by radical lesbian feminist Jean O'Leary, who accused Rivera of mocking womanhood. Rivera forced her way on to the stage and delivered one of her most famous speeches, referred to as "Y'all better quiet down," where she called out the whiteness and privilege of the movement (and the audience), and how that made them blind to the struggles of underprivileged, gender non-conforming, queer people of colour. Rivera was initially booed by the crowd, although after her impassioned speech about both her own experiences and those of the people whose rights she was fighting for, as well as everything she had sacrificed for the movement, the crowd began to cheer.

However, despite her rousing speech, Rivera's spirit was broken by O'Leary's actions that day. She disbanded STAR and attempted suicide – although luckily Johnson found her in time to save her – and abstained from activism for two decades. However, after Johnson's death, Rivera returned to activism in 1993, rejoining the gay rights movement and reforming STAR.

Rivera fought aggressively for queer visibility in her final years before she died in 2002. Her ashes reside at the Metropolitan Community Church of New York, where she had attended services and worked in the food pantry. The Church renamed its homeless shelter for LGBTQ youth Sylvia's Place in her memory.

THEIR AWESOME ACHIEVEMENTS

➜ Helped with the instigation and continued momentum of the Stonewall uprising.

➜ Became one of America's first transgender rights activists.

➜ Fought for and achieved the Sexual Orientation Non-Discrimination Act of New York, preventing barriers being put up for the LGBTQ community in work, housing, services and more.

➜ Fought for a similar bill with the New York City Gay Rights Bill.

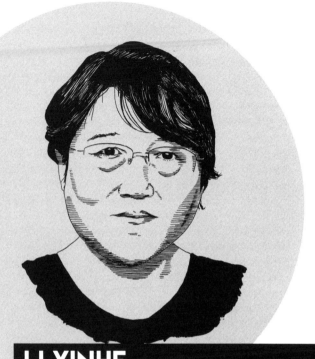

LI YINHE

1952–PRESENT

SUPERPOWERS

Equal marriage and LGBTQ rights activist, China's first sexologist.

THEIR INCREDIBLE STORY

As an academic and an activist for LGBTQ rights in China, Li Yinhe has spent most of her career advocating for changes in the laws that target sexual minorities alongside the LGBTQ community.

Yinhe graduated from Shanxi University with a degree in history, before achieving her doctorate in sociology from the University of Pittsburgh in 1998, where she established herself as an academic. Since then, Yinhe has dedicated her work to fighting for equality in China. In 2000, as the National People's Congress prepared to revise marriage laws, Yinhe made her first proposal to legalize same-sex marriage in China. Her argument was dismissed by the Congress and she was told that China did not need to lead the world in this regard.

Yinhe's philosophies are not popular in China and she has been subjected to much criticism and aggression for her work. On her blog about same-sex marriage – found on Chinese blogging platform Weibo – death threats are sadly not uncommon. However, Yinhe takes these in her stride and continues her important work – she simply acknowledges that people get emotional and passionate about these topics and carries on.

Criticisms against Yinhe have occasionally presented her with an opportunity to educate. In 2014, she decided to go public about her relationship after she was accused of being a lesbian, following the revelation that her partner was a transgender man. Yinhe felt the need to clarify her sexuality, not because she harboured any disrespect for lesbians, but simply because she was not one to suffer the spread of misinformation.

The transgender community in China, as in many countries, faces a lot of discrimination and misunderstanding, so Yinhe used the opportunity to shine light on this area of society. Yinhe was clear on her partner's identity as a man and that she was heterosexual. In her response, Yinhe sparked a conversation that had previously been non-existent in mainstream China.

Yinhe also fights for the abolition of laws that criminalize group sex and prostitution. Sex is not a widely discussed topic in China, so Yinhe has been a pioneer in the conversation. To that end, she is often described as "China's first sexologist", and a pioneer of gender studies in mainland China. She has also been very critical of the country's introduction of laws to ban LGBTQ content from the internet, with the regulation banning any display of "abnormal sexual behaviours". Yinhe has warned that this could lead to all art being censored and queer resources being restricted to those most in need. She continues to encourage the conversation on and fight for the rights of the LGBTQ community in China.

THEIR AWESOME ACHIEVEMENTS

➔ Won the China Rainbow Media Awards Special Contribution Award in 2011.

➔ Strongly and proudly supports the LGBTQ community of China, undeterred by online death threats.

➔ Creates conversations on gender, sexuality and sex in China – previously undiscussed topics.

➔ Continues to speak out against anti-LGBTQ laws and any prejudice in China.

➔ Campaigns for LGBTQ civil and equal rights in China.

"HOMOSEXUAL PEOPLE SHOULD BE ENTITLED TO THE SAME RIGHTS AS ANY CITIZEN OF THE PEOPLE'S REPUBLIC OF CHINA TO FREELY CHOOSE THEIR SEXUAL PARTNER AND TO GET MARRIED."

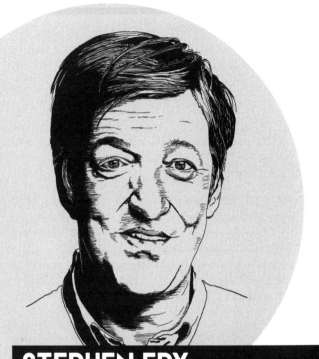

STEPHEN FRY

1957–PRESENT

SUPERPOWERS

The man with all the facts, LGBTQ rights activist, sharer of worldwide LGBTQ experiences and struggles.

THEIR INCREDIBLE STORY

Stephen Fry is best known for hosting British television show *QI* and for his roles in TV and film, as well as for his work as an LGBTQ activist. In his early years, Fry tried to stay private about his sexuality, often struggling at the hands of the British press. More recently he has been more open after he realized how important it is to the queer community to see high-profile LGBTQ people in public.

In recent years, Fry has worked to broaden understanding of the struggles and experiences of the LGBTQ community worldwide. In his 2013 documentary, *Stephen Fry: Out There*, he travelled to Uganda, where the government was debating outlawing homosexuality (they have since introduced a law that sentences homosexuals to death). Fry also travelled to parts of the USA where he explored the impact of conversion therapy. In Brazil, where he revealed that one gay person is murdered every 36 hours, he interviewed anti-gay politician Jair Bolsonaro. Bolsonaro – who is now the president of Brazil – was adamant that there was no homophobia in Brazil, and that homosexual deaths were often due to drug problems, prostitution or domestic violence. Bolsonaro said that teaching young children about homosexuality would cause them to become gay. In addition to opposing these views, Fry took particular issue with Bolsonaro's statement that homosexuality is "not normal", using the example of the hundreds of species of animals on earth that exhibit homosexuality and the only one to exhibit homophobia is the human race – and that we are the anomaly in this case. Fry kept his cool during the interview, asserting that no gay person, himself included, would want to "turn" anyone gay as part of an agenda, and any fear that a homosexual life is an unhappy one can be attributed to homophobia still existing so openly in the world.

In his travels to India, Fry highlighted the prejudice faced by the transgender and intersex community (known as the hijras) and the struggles they experience; this community had historically been celebrated in India prior to British colonization. When the British arrived, the hijras were ostracized, the impact of which could still be felt at the time of Fry's travels, with the community living in slums and many scraping by through sex work – which sadly led to further struggles due to HIV/AIDS.

Fry revealed during his time in India that prior to colonization, India had always been very open in regard to sexuality and gender. In fact, the first family Fry spoke to during his visit were very accepting of their son being gay. Fry even discovered a shop proudly displaying rainbow flags and much to his delight discovered the owners were openly gay.

Today Fry continues to share LGBTQ experiences and raise awareness of the issues faced by the community, taking an active role in debates to ensure the fight for queer rights remains progressive.

THEIR AWESOME ACHIEVEMENTS

→ Awarded honorary doctorates from the universities of Dundee and Sussex, an honorary degree from Anglia Ruskin University and made an honorary fellow of Cardiff University.

→ Declared Mind Champion of the Year in 2007 and in 2011 became the mental health charity's president.

→ Awarded numerous BAFTAs for his television work and in 2007, the documentary about his mental health *The Secret Life of the Manic Depressive* won a BAFTA for Best Factual Series.

→ Awarded a Rose d'Or for Best Game Show Host for *QI*.

→ Honoured with the Outstanding Lifetime Achievement Award in Cultural Humanism by the Humanist Chaplaincy at Harvard University, the Harvard Secular Society and the American Humanist Association.

→ Brought awareness and visibility to the issues faced by the LGBTQ community in various places across the world with his documentary *Out There*, often putting himself at risk in being an openly gay man in these locations.

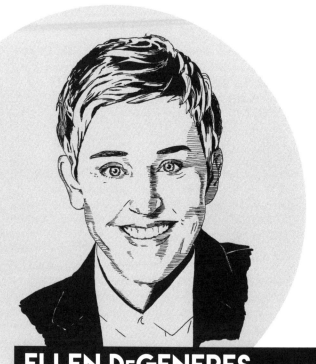

ELLEN DeGENERES

1958—PRESENT

SUPERPOWERS

Beloved talk show host, queer visibility advocate, changer of hearts and minds.

THEIR INCREDIBLE STORY

Beloved actor and comedian turned LGBTQ icon Ellen DeGeneres made her mark as the first lesbian to play an openly lesbian character on television when she portrayed the titular character in *Ellen*.

In 1997 a *TIME Magazine* cover featured DeGeneres with the words, "Yep, I'm Gay." No longer wanting to live her life ashamed of her sexuality, DeGeneres made the decision to appear in the magazine and come out publicly. Later that year, DeGeneres would reaffirm her coming out story on *The Oprah Winfrey Show*. At a similar time, her character, Ellen Morgan, on the ABC Network sitcom *Ellen*, also came out in 'The Puppy Episode'.

DeGeneres became a pioneer in LGBTQ rights by coming out. In the 1990s, LGBTQ rights were still lacking and visibility of the queer community was minimal. Sadly, however, *Ellen* was cancelled a year after 'The Puppy Episode'. DeGeneres received hate mail and threats leading up to the episode and afterward, and was briefly snubbed by Hollywood. However, the studio and DeGeneres also received letters from people thanking her for her influence and bravely being so public with coming out – some even said it had kept them from suicide. By coming out both in reality and portraying a lesbian character on television, DeGeneres showed that LGBTQ people do exist and that their existence was not something to be feared or hated.

As the host of her own talk show, *The Ellen DeGeneres Show*, DeGeneres has gone above and beyond in the fight for LGBTQ visibility. The long-running show has hosted many queer guests and needless to say her own presence has done a lot to normalize the existence of LGBTQ lives. The show has also contributed to important queer discussions, such as transgender experiences when Laverne Cox made an appearance. Actor Asia Kate Dillon appeared on the show and discussed their non-binary gender identity, furthering the conversation around gender in the media.

In a 2008 episode of *The Ellen DeGeneres Show*, DeGeneres announced her engagement to Portia de Rossi. Since their marriage, de Rossi has made several appearances on DeGeneres' show. In a particularly heartwarming surprise appearance on DeGeneres' 60th birthday episode, de Rossi surprised her by announcing plans to build the Ellen DeGeneres Campus of the Dian Fossey Gorilla Fund – a cause close to DeGeneres' heart as an animal rights advocate. The love between DeGeneres and de Rossi was always unquestionable in these appearances, proving that queer love is as valid and powerful as any love.

Even President Barack Obama appeared on DeGeneres' talk show. In a touching moment, he thanked DeGeneres for helping him improve LGBTQ rights for US citizens. Because of her ability to change the hearts and minds of people, and for her activism in LGBTQ rights and visibility, DeGeneres was awarded the Presidential Medal of Freedom in 2016.

THEIR AWESOME ACHIEVEMENTS

→ Was the first lesbian actor to play an openly lesbian character on television.

→ Endured public hate and temporary snubbing from Hollywood by coming out, limiting her career and causing her to become depressed.

→ Became a visible icon for the LGBTQ community, empowering many to live their queer lives without shame.

→ Began a successful talk show that has done amazing things for queer visibility.

→ Is now a widely loved public figure, known for her warm personality, acting and comedic talents, and being out and proud of her identity.

→ Awarded the Presidential Medal of Freedom in 2016.

→ Won so many Daytime Emmy Awards (almost 60) for *The Ellen DeGeneres Show* that it surpassed *The Oprah Winfrey Show*.

→ Awarded the Mark Twain Prize for American Humor.

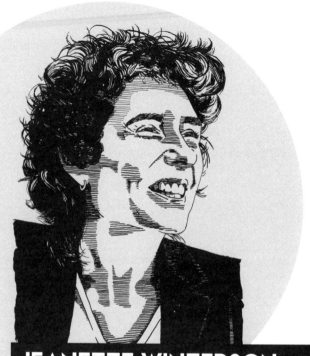

JEANETTE WINTERSON

1959–PRESENT

SUPERPOWERS

Writer, feminist, champion of lesbian visibility, experience sharer.

THEIR INCREDIBLE STORY

Winterson left home at 16 years old. Upon leaving, her mother (whom she refers to as "Mrs Winterson" in articles she writes for *The Guardian*) asked her a question that would later inspire a memoir, "Why be happy when you could be normal?" Winterson's family were strict evangelical Christians and unfortunately, her first love did not sit right with their beliefs, because her first love was another girl.

She went on to study at St Catherine's College Oxford and from there moved to London and wrote her first book, *Oranges Are Not the Only Fruit*, which was published in 1985. The semi-autobiographical book told a coming-of-age story following a girl, also named Jeanette, growing up in her hometown of Accrington, Lancashire. Jeanette is a lesbian and finds herself attracted to another girl, however, the local religious community – her mother's friends – subject her and her partner to exorcisms. When the novel was published, Winterson recalled receiving an angry note from her mother due to the similarities to Winterson's experiences growing up.

Since its publication, *Oranges Are Not the Only Fruit* has sometimes been referred to by academics and educators as a "lesbian novel". Winterson rejects the label, expressing her dislike for the idea that "straight fiction" is for everyone but novels and media with gay characters or any queer experience are only for queer people.

Winterson has written several books that explore gender, sexuality and the boundaries of physicality and imagination, including *Sexing the Cherry* and *Written on the Body*. *Oranges Are Not the Only Fruit* was also adapted for television by Winterson herself in 1990, allowing the story to reach a wider audience. Many books later, Winterson would go on to write her memoir in 2011, the aforementioned *Why Be Happy When You Could Be Normal?* Though she is married herself, Winterson rejects the idea that the institution of marriage should be something women are expected to strive for, as is often portrayed in the media. When she married Susie Orbach in 2015, Winterson wrote her own vows that better reflected her views on partnership, taking issue with the "for richer, for poorer" in standard wedding vows. To her, the usual wedding vows spoke more of a life sentence than any kind of liberation from loneliness or celebration of each other's love. Instead, Winterson's vows included the following promises: "I promise to respect you: the you that is you; the you that is not me; the you that is not us. I promise to stand by you in the world. I promise to delight in you." Winterson later had her vows written by calligrapher Stephen Raw and hung them on her bedroom wall – she likes to sleep next to her promises.

THEIR AWESOME ACHIEVEMENTS

→ Awarded an OBE and CBE for Services to Literature in 2006 and 2018.

→ Won Lambda Literary awards for *Written on the Body* in 1994's Lesbian Fiction category and *Why Be Happy When You Could Be Normal?* in 2013's Lesbian Memoir or Biography category.

→ Received the E. M. Forster Award for *Sexing the Cherry* in 1989.

→ Became a professor of creative writing at the University of Manchester in 2012.

→ Became a Fellow of the Royal Society of Literature and made the BBC's 100 Women List in 2016.

→ Shared her queer experiences, as well as her struggles with religion and complex family relationships, in her first semi-autobiographical book, *Oranges Are Not the Only Fruit* in 1985. The novel won the Whitbread Award for a first novel.

"I AM A WRITER WHO HAPPENS TO LOVE WOMEN. I AM NOT A LESBIAN WHO HAPPENS TO WRITE."

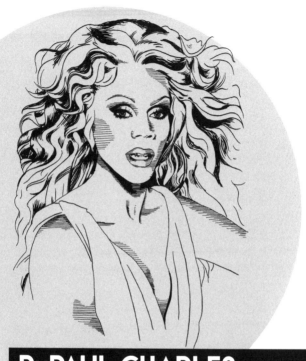

RuPAUL CHARLES

1960–PRESENT

SUPERPOWERS

Drag queen, supermodel, actor, singer, author.

THEIR INCREDIBLE STORY

The "drag queen supermodel of the world" RuPaul Charles (or just Ru, if you're on good terms) is known predominantly as the most commercially successful drag queen in America. RuPaul has done it all: acting, singing, modelling, writing and even producing his own highly successful TV show – *RuPaul's Drag Race*. As a black, gay man in a wig, the success he has achieved is no mean feat.

In the 1980s, RuPaul co-produced and starred in *RuPaul Is: Starbooty!* The extremely low-budget film trilogy harkened back to 1960s blacksploitation movies, in which RuPaul portrays ex-model turned US federal agent Starbooty going on crime-fighting adventures, having the odd romance along the way. The trilogy was distributed on cheaply manufactured cassette tapes, handed out in clubs and on the streets.

RuPaul's music career started with his first album in 1993, *Supermodel of the World*, with the music video for "Supermodel (You Better Work)" becoming an unexpected success on MTV. A couple of singles later and RuPaul had signed modelling contracts for MAC Cosmetics, landing him on billboards in full drag. *The RuPaul Show* and an autobiography followed not long afterward. In 2007, *Starrbooty* returned – this time with a much higher budget (and a new spelling) – and RuPaul again took on the titular role. The new film combined elements of the three originals, however *Starrbooty* featured an all-new story rather than being a full remake. RuPaul also presented a much more feminine Starrbooty this time around, with body padding, wigs and all.

In 2008, RuPaul changed the world of drag forever, when he created *RuPaul's Drag Race*. The show brought a group of drag queens from across America together to compete for the title of America's Next Drag Superstar. With each year a new season brings in a new selection of queens, boosting the careers of the majority of the contestants whether they win or not.

While RuPaul had reached an admirable level of success, *RuPaul's Drag Race* is what really made him a household name. The show allowed drag to break in to the mainstream and its popularity has even led to an overseas spin-off show, *Drag Race Thailand*, with upcoming versions rumoured in both the UK and Brazil.

By sharing his success with *Drag Race*, RuPaul provided a platform for a whole new generation of drag queens. Today the show still continues to further discussions on gender, with many transgender contestants going on to take the conversation to wider audiences.

"WHATEVER PEOPLE THINK OF ME IS NONE OF MY BUSINESS."

THEIR AWESOME ACHIEVEMENTS

→ Became the world's first drag queen supermodel.

→ One of the first openly gay talk show hosts on US national television with *The RuPaul Show*.

→ Used his platform to discuss black empowerment, female empowerment, misogyny and other "taboo" topics publicly in the 1990s.

→ Was the first drag queen to secure a major cosmetics contract with MAC Cosmetics, where he raises money for the MAC AIDS Fund.

→ Boasts an impressive discography of 11 studio albums.

→ Won the GLAAD Media Vito Russo Award in 1999 for promoting equality in the LGBTQ community.

→ Created *RuPaul's Drag Race*, giving drag queens across America the chance to achieve new heights of fame and success.

→ Won three Primetime Emmy Awards for Outstanding Host on *RuPaul's Drag Race*.

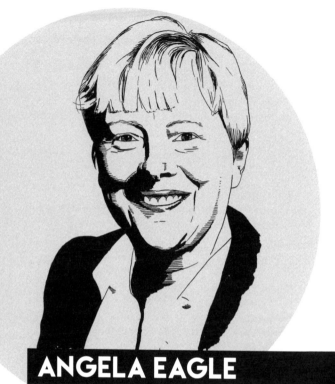

ANGELA EAGLE

1961–PRESENT

SUPERPOWERS

Openly gay minister, politician, LGBTQ rights activist.

THEIR INCREDIBLE STORY

Angela Eagle is a British politician and has been an active member of the UK's Labour Party since 1992. Eagle made history when she came out as gay in 1997, making her the first female MP to do so while in office.

As a queer politician, Eagle understands the importance of visibility. She came out in a newspaper interview, publicly revealing her sexuality in solidarity with the LGBTQ community of the UK, which was still suffering due to the Section 28 clause banning the "promotion" of homosexuality and subjecting queer people to heavy prejudice. Eagle would remain the only out lesbian politician in Westminster for 10 years.

Eagle was a part of the standing committee that saw the introduction of the Civil Partnership Act in 2004. In all but name civil partnerships granted same-sex couples in the UK many of the same rights as married couples. Four years after the introduction, Eagle became the first MP to enter into a civil partnership. Since then, marriage equality in the UK has been introduced, with people now criticizing the fact that civil partnerships were offered in the first place as opposed to equal marriage for all.

As a queer woman, Eagle has faced discrimination on many levels during her time in Westminster. When David Cameron became Prime Minister, Eagle called him out on several issues, the first during a row on NHS reforms during which Cameron told

Eagle to "calm down, dear". He was accused of sexism, with Eagle saying, "I don't think a modern man would have expressed himself that way." Eagle was also the target of homophobic abuse during her run for leadership of the Labour Party, against Jeremy Corbyn, in 2016. She spoke to the press about receiving many abusive, homophobic and frightening messages, including death threats, during this time – and her office was vandalized by someone throwing a brick through the window. One man was convicted for sending death threats to Eagle and the whole case highlighted just how quickly queer politicians can be faced with homophobic abuse – abuse that Eagle said she would no longer tolerate. Eagle did find an ally in Corbyn at this time, expressing gratitude that he had joined her in meetings to investigate the abuse against her.

During Eagle's time in government, the Labour Party has taken strides to improve the rights of the LGBTQ community, achievements that Eagle expressed pride in during LGBT History Month 2018. The party has seen the age of sexual consent for homosexuals equalized with heterosexuals, LGBTQ people given the chance to serve openly in the armed forces, discrimination against LGBTQ people for goods and services outlawed and sexual offence legislation no longer specifically discriminating against gay men.

Eagle continues to remind us that the rights of the LGBTQ community in the UK have been hard fought and that we must remain vigilant to keep up that progress.

THEIR AWESOME ACHIEVEMENTS

→ Became the first openly lesbian government minister elected in the UK, in 1992.

→ Was the first government minister to enter into a civil partnership, in 2008.

→ Held a role as part of the committee that introduced civil partnerships as an alternative to marriage in the UK before same-sex marriage was introduced.

→ Took part in LGBTQ equality reforms including equal age of consent, the right to serve in the armed forces, outlawing discrimination for business, housing or services and discrimination against gay men in sexual offences legislation.

"PROGRESS HAS BEEN MADE, BUT WE HAVE TO REMEMBER THAT THINGS CAN GO BACKWARD IF WE ARE NOT VIGILANT."

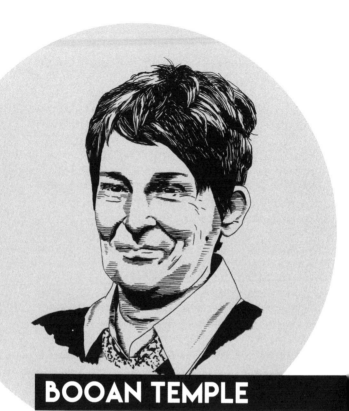

BOOAN TEMPLE

DOB UNKNOWN–PRESENT

SUPERPOWERS

"Stop Section 28!", LGBTQ rights activist.

THEIR INCREDIBLE STORY

Booan Temple has managed to mostly avoid fame, but her actions have made her a queer icon nonetheless. The significance of her protests to the Section 28 clause in UK law cannot be understated. Temple's story as an icon began shortly before the introduction of Section 28 in 1988, when the proposal began to gain traction. The Section 28 clause of the Local Government Act 1988 would forbid local authorities and education institutions from distributing any information that would "promote" homosexuality. Any education in the UK on LGBTQ issues would cease and queer youth would be left without any resources to educate themselves, or be educated, on queer identities. Though homosexuality had been decriminalized in the UK in 1967, attitudes toward the LGBTQ community had not improved. In the 1980s, homosexuality was met with more hatred from society amid the AIDS crisis and Temple felt unsafe in public. The UK's Conservative Party was attacking homosexuality and its "promotion" to young people as immoral – believing that teaching children and young people about homosexuality would encourage them to be homosexual.

Temple, like many others, recognized the danger Section 28 posed to the already vulnerable LGBTQ community, with the UK already such a hostile environment. Taking away education about the LGBTQ community would worsen these attitudes and leave young queer people more vulnerable – ignorance would breed intolerance.

In response to Section 28, protest groups formed across the UK, even seeing famed actor Ian McKellen join in. Temple realized the protests weren't getting enough coverage to make an impact, so she sought to become the news. This meant actually getting on the news and in May 1988, Temple made that happen. Along with a group of lesbian activists, she stormed into the BBC Television Centre studios as a news broadcast was going out live. Temple recalls how the place went mad and she was violently subdued. One member of her group managed to handcuff herself to a camera, causing further disruption. Temple shouted as the broadcast went out to the country, "Stop Section 28!" The protest gained huge media coverage and empowered young LGBTQ people.

Temple was invited back to the BBC 30 years later to tell her story and talk about how things have changed for the LGBTQ community. She recognized that while things have improved, there is still homophobia as a result of Section 28 and that the LGBTQ community needs to be in solidarity with smaller communities worldwide. In 2003, Section 28 was successfully repealed, but without Booan Temple it might still be around today.

THEIR AWESOME ACHIEVEMENTS

→ Campaigned against the introduction of Section 28 into British law despite threats to her safety.

→ Successfully broke into the BBC during a news broadcast to protest Section 28.

→ Inspired a generation of young queer people watching to protest against Section 28 and any anti-LGBTQ laws.

→ Continues to speak out for LGBTQ equality and solidarity worldwide.

"I, AND MANY OF MY LOVED ONES, HAD BEEN ATTACKED IN THE STREET. THERE WAS AN ATMOSPHERE THAT 'THE OTHER' NEEDED TO BE ERADICATED AND I THINK THE LGBT COMMUNITY WAS SEEN AS A THREAT TO THE INSTITUTION OF THE FAMILY. SECTION 28 WAS PART OF THAT."

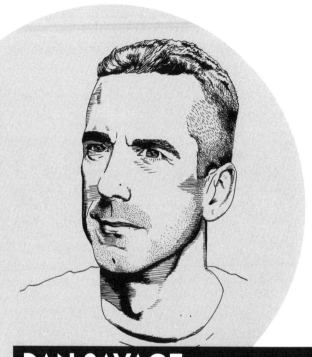

DAN SAVAGE

1969–PRESENT

SUPERPOWERS

LGBTQ political activist, queer writer, founder of the It Gets Better Project.

THEIR INCREDIBLE STORY

Journalist Dan Savage is an LGBTQ activist and founder of social justice movement, the It Gets Better Project. Although he sometimes finds himself at the centre of controversy due to his occasionally sharp comments, his work as an advocate for LGBTQ rights cannot be understated.

Savage began his career as a journalist with a simple offhand comment. Tim Keck, co-founder of *The Onion*, had launched an alternative news source called *The Stranger* and Savage advised him to include an advice column – because everyone claims to hate them but loves to read them. Savage ended up writing that advice column for *The Stranger*.

The advice column 'Savage Love', which focused on sex advice, started in 1991 and has featured in many (mostly free) newspapers as well as *The Stranger* across the US, Canada, Europe and Asia. In a 2006 interview, Savage said he began the column with the purpose of mocking heterosexuals after seeing many straight advice columnists' clueless responses to letters from gay people. However, Savage does answer the questions he receives with honesty and integrity, often providing sound advice that ranges from short and snappy to lengthy responses.

The column is also well known for its interesting language, with Savage coining words and expressions to summarize situations and sexual acts. These include words like "monogamish", referencing couples who are perceived to be monogamous though are not fully so. He has also encouraged readers to coin similar terms, such as "pegging" – the act of a woman penetrating her male partner using a strap-on dildo. This has sometimes resulted in controversy, for example he has been criticized for attempting to reclaim offensive words, by initially encouraging readers to address their letter "Hey faggot". The reclaiming of the slur – the act of an oppressed group using a word used to oppress them, usually as a term of endearment – is still a hotly debated topic.

Savage started the It Gets Better Project in response to the death of teen Billy Lucas, who committed suicide as a result of bullying for his perceived sexuality. The project saw many queer celebrities and allies sharing their experiences of being bullied and speaking out against the idea that bullying is a "rite of passage" that everyone should have to endure. President Barack Obama was one of many to lend his voice and support to the project.

It Gets Better continues to make waves today, with many still using the project to speak out against LGBTQ bullying. The project has spread worldwide, prompting many other countries to create their own similar initiatives to put an end to LGBTQ bullying.

THEIR AWESOME ACHIEVEMENTS

→ Started a worldwide anti-bullying queer movement with the It Gets Better Project.

→ Won the Webby Award for Special Achievement for It Gets Better in 2011.

→ Awarded the Anthony Giffard Make the Change Award for It Gets Better in 2011.

→ Given the Bonham Centre Award by The Mark S. Bonham Centre for Sexual Diversity Studies at the University of Toronto for It Gets Better in 2013.

→ Awarded Humanist of the Year by The American Humanist Association in 2013.

"HOW CAN YOU TELL SOMEBODY WHO IS PURSUING HAPPINESS THAT THEY'RE SOMEHOW NOT AMERICAN WHEN THAT WAS THE VERY FIRST PROMISE THAT AMERICA MADE?"

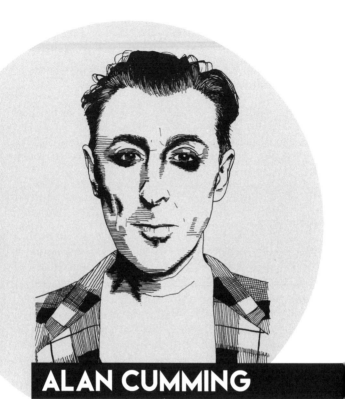

ALAN CUMMING

1965–PRESENT

SUPERPOWERS

*Actor, bisexuality visibility advocate,
equal marriage rights activist.*

THEIR INCREDIBLE STORY

Stage and film actor, director and writer Alan Cumming is most known for his acting roles. However, he also works tirelessly for the LGBTQ community, pursuing equal and civil rights on both sides of the Atlantic.

The Scottish actor is most widely recognized for his film roles in *Goldeneye*, *Spy Kids* and the X-Men franchise. He even made an appearance in *Spice World* alongside the legendary Spice Girls.

Cumming is open about his sexuality as a bisexual man and has long fought against bi-erasure (the removal or re-explanation of bisexuality in history and the media). Cumming talks in great detail about his sexuality, being clear that although he has been in a long-term relationship with a man, he still experiences attraction to women. Having previously been married to Hilary Lyon and now married to Grant Shaffer, it's fair to say he recognizes the importance of equality. As a member of the Gay and Lesbian Alliance Against Defamation (GLAAD) and being involved in the Human Rights Campaign, Cumming puts in a lot of time campaigning for marriage equality and other civil rights for the LGBTQ community. In an interview with *Instinct Magazine*, Cumming talked about how he believes that, despite the progress that has been made, there is still a long way to go for LGBTQ rights and until laws are equal, prejudice will pervade in society.

Cumming is also a strong supporter of many AIDS charities. He has worked with the American Foundation for AIDS Research and Broadway Care/Equity Fights AIDS – recording a duet of 'Baby, It's Cold Outside' with Liza Minelli for a Christmas album, with the profits going to the Broadway Cares/Equity Fights AIDS fund. Along with the Broadway cast of *Cabaret*, Cumming also collected donations for the same fund during the Gypsy of the Year fundraising season. In interviews he has often discussed his solidarity with those living with HIV/AIDS in order to raise awareness of their impact on the LGBTQ community.

In his film and stage roles, Cumming is known to portray a diverse series of characters. In television he played a political role in *The Good Wife*, and on stage he has donned stockings and rouge for his Broadway role in *Cabaret*. More recently, he plays a leading role in *Instinct* as a gay character, making his the first openly gay lead in an American network television drama series. This represents a huge shift in the depiction of LGBTQ characters in mainstream media, with Cumming being the one to open people's minds.

THEIR AWESOME ACHIEVEMENTS

→ Received an Olivier Award for Comedy Performance of the Year for his role in the National Theatre's *Accidental Death of an Anarchist* in 1991, a British Comedy Award for Best TV Comedy Newcomer for *Bernard and the Genie* in 1992 and Best Actor for *Prague* at the Atlantic Film Festival in 1992.

→ Winner of multiple awards, including: HRC Humanitarian Award, GLAAD Media Vito Russo Award, New York Free Press Award, Tony Award, and Artistic Achievement Award from the Philadelphia International Gay & Lesbian Film Festival, and was inducted into the Vanity Fair Hall of Fame.

→ Raised awareness and funds for Broadway Cares/Equity Fights AIDS fund in solidarity with those living with HIV/AIDS.

→ Campaigns for marriage equality across the the UK and US.

"IT IS NOT HARD TO FEEL LIKE AN OUTSIDER. I THINK WE HAVE ALL FELT LIKE THAT AT ONE TIME OR ANOTHER."

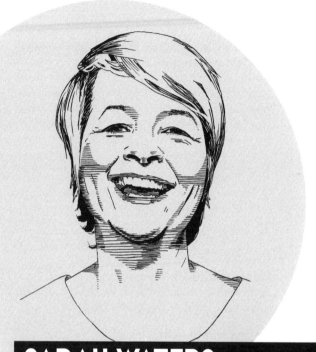

SARAH WATERS

1966–PRESENT

SUPERPOWERS

Lesbian writer, academic, proud author with a lesbian agenda.

THEIR INCREDIBLE STORY

Sarah Waters is well known for her novels, which feature lesbian protagonists, and has been clear about the lesbian agenda within her books, writing for both visibility and to normalize LGBTQ lives.

Waters was an academic prior to her novelist career, achieving a BA, MA and PhD at the University of Kent, Lancaster University and Queen Mary University of London respectively. Waters went straight from her doctoral thesis to writing her first novel. She was inspired to the title *Tipping the Velvet* while researching nineteenth-century pornography. Research and authenticity is a key part of Waters' novels – something she enjoys as an academic – because of the historical setting of the majority of her books.

All but one of her novels (*The Night Watch*) have featured lesbian protagonists and she said she missed writing lesbian characters while working on it. She says that the sexualities of her characters are incidental and that they simply reflect her own experience.

Waters found writing her first book to be exhilarating, especially being able to focus on queer characters. Just in revealing the plot, she was outing herself as a lesbian. She hadn't expected *Tipping the Velvet* to be such a success, particularly with straight readers, and the book was adapted into a television series for the BBC in 2002, reaching an even wider audience. Waters' third novel, *Fingersmith*, received similar attention from the BBC in 2005 and was adapted into South Korean film *The Handmaiden* in 2016.

The importance of Waters' work cannot be understated. Her novels have told queer stories via the mainstream, giving visibility to the LGBTQ community. Thanks to the popularity of her novels, with the help of television adaptations and on the merit of the source materials, Waters' queer stories have reached a wide audience, furthering her self-proclaimed lesbian agenda.

"RESPECT YOUR CHARACTERS, EVEN THE MINOR ONES. IN ART, AS IN LIFE, EVERYONE IS THE HERO OF THEIR OWN PARTICULAR STORY."

THEIR AWESOME ACHIEVEMENTS

→ Listed in the 20 Best of Young British Writers by Granta Magazine and won Author of the Year at the British Book Awards in 2003.

→ Won Writer of the Year at the Stonewall Awards in 2006 and 2009, as well as receiving various literary awards too numerous to mention.

→ Proudly writes with a lesbian agenda in her novels, never shying away from queer eroticism and experiences in her work. She continues to push queer themes in her fiction, giving queer readers stories they can relate to and an eye-opening experience to all readers.

→ Unafraid to find and write queer stories in period pieces, set in times that were widely considered to be quite heterosexual.

"WHY DO GENTLEMEN'S VOICES CARRY SO CLEARLY, WHEN WOMEN'S ARE SO EASILY STIFLED?"

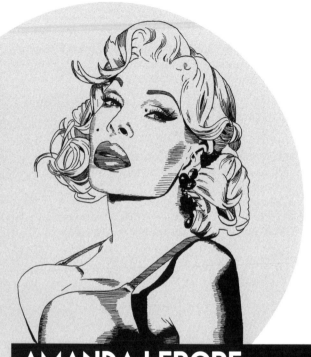

AMANDA LEPORE

1967–PRESENT

SUPERPOWERS

Queen of the Club, transgender icon, photographic muse, prominent nightlife figure.

THEIR INCREDIBLE STORY

The original Queen of the Club, Amanda Lepore made a name for herself as a photographic muse, singer, model and party-goer in New York City, with a great head for business. Being vocal about her transgender identity, Lepore's high profile does a lot for transgender visibility.

"Ever since I can remember, I knew I was a girl," Lepore said in 2007. "I couldn't understand why my parents were dressing me up in boys' clothing. I thought they were insane."

Growing up in New Jersey, Lepore's school forbade her from wearing a girl's uniform, denying her identity, which led to her being privately schooled so she could begin her journey in transitioning. At 15 years old, she designed costumes for the dancers of a local strip club and was paid by the dancers in female hormones.

After meeting her first husband, who accepted her transitioning, she began the physical process with the help of her husband's supportive parents. However, when her husband became abusive – to the point where he would not allow her to leave the house – and changed his tune about her transition, Lepore was forced to file a restraining order and divorce him.

Lepore rose to fame in the 1990s after moving to New York City, where she hosted a club night in Bowery Bar and attempted to establish herself as a nightlife figure. There she met photographer David LaChapelle, became his muse and appeared in his work regularly. Lepore went on to appear in many magazines, even French *Playboy*, and music videos by artists such as Grace Jones and Elton John. Although attitudes to LGBTQ individuals left a lot to be desired, Lepore's identity never held her back – she was championing transgender visibility.

Lepore's career continues to span the worlds of film and music and she remains a popular nightlife figure. She appeared in documentary *Party Monster* and made a cameo in the film of the same name, based on club kid culture. She is proud and vocal about her identity and in turn raises the visibility of the transgender community.

"I REALLY ASSOCIATE GLAMOUR WITH BEING HAPPY. IF YOU PUT ON HIGH HEELS AND LIPSTICK OR GET A NEW OUTFIT, YOU FEEL GREAT. IT'S A CELEBRATION OF LOVING YOURSELF AND THE WHOLE RITUAL OF IT IS SO GREAT."

THEIR AWESOME ACHIEVEMENTS

➔ Worked tirelessly to make a name for herself in the New York City club scene and succeeded in becoming a nightlife figure.

➔ Promotes visibility of the transgender community and to that end is very open about her identity.

➔ Became the muse of photographer David LaChapelle and worked with many other photographers including Terry Richardson and Ruben van Schalm.

➔ Appeared in numerous advertising campaigns, including a Sergio K fashion campaign, Behance, MAC Cosmetics and Armani Jeans, to name a few.

➔ Appeared in music videos for big-name artists such as Elton John, The Dandy Warhols, Grace Jones and Cazwell. Cazwell has also written many singles for Lepore.

➔ Released her debut album, *I... Amanda Lepore* in 2011.

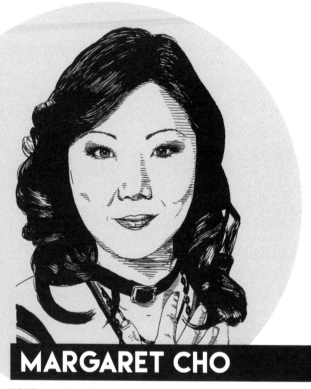

MARGARET CHO

1968–PRESENT

SUPERPOWERS

*Bisexual visibility advocate, voting activist,
queer comedian, sex positive.*

THEIR INCREDIBLE STORY

Cho's career as a stand-up comedian started close to home, with a few shows in a local club near her parents' bookstore in San Francisco. Garnering a taste for performance, she toured the comedy club circuit developing her material and soon started making appearances on television shows with a few small roles here and there. Eventually, Cho was approached by the network ABC, which devised the show *All-American Girl* based on her stand-up routine.

Airing in 2014, *All-American Girl* featured an East Asian family as its central characters and had the potential to be groundbreaking. Sadly, it proved problematic both with East Asian audiences, who would criticize the show over stereotypical portrayals, and Cho, who struggled with the portrayal of her character. Producers would at times tell her to "be more Asian" and at others that she was "not Asian enough".

After one season *All-American Girl* was cancelled, which led to Cho suffering from depression and experiencing problems with addiction. Looking back, Cho has expressed regret at the stereotypical depictions of the characters in the show.

Cho eventually bounced back and returned to stand-up comedy. In her one-woman show, *I'm the One That I Want*, Cho would joke about her struggles with depression, race and sexuality. The show won her the New York Magazine's Performance of the Year award. Cho was back on her game.

Cho has faced some challenges when it comes to her bisexuality: she has faced bi-erasure and has struggled to get people to accept her identity, especially in relationships. Cho has also expressed an internal struggle with the label, expressing concern at the implication that there are only two genders, particularly with the rise in prominence of the identity pansexual (a sexual or romantic attraction to people of any gender). However, Cho has said she believes bisexual is the right label for her.

Cho's openness about her experiences as a queer woman of colour continues to normalize the experiences of the LGBTQ community worldwide. Cho is also very sex positive and has been open about her experiences with polyamory, further normalizing non-heteronormative experiences.

"SOMETIMES WHEN WE ARE GENEROUS IN SMALL, BARELY DETECTABLE WAYS IT CAN CHANGE SOMEONE ELSE'S LIFE FOREVER."

THEIR AWESOME ACHIEVEMENTS

→ Champion of bisexual visibility in the fight against bi-erasure.

→ Fighter for the rights of queer women of colour.

→ Openly discusses, raises awareness of and normalizes practices such as polyamory, sexual kinks and fetishes, and general sex positivity.

→ Received the American Comedy Award for Best Female Comedian in 1994 and the GLAAD Golden Gate Award in 2000.

→ Awarded the Justice in Action Award by the Asian American Legal Defense and Education Fund for her use of comedy to challenge racism, sexism and social injustice in 2003.

→ Received the First Amendment Award from the American Civil Liberties Union in 2004 and won an Intrepid Award from the National Organization for Women.

→ Won the Asian Excellence Award for Outstanding Comedian in 2007.

"JUST BECAUSE YOU ARE BLIND AND UNABLE TO SEE MY BEAUTY DOESN'T MEAN IT DOES NOT EXIST."

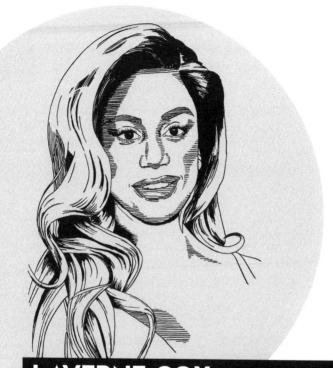

LAVERNE COX

1972–PRESENT

SUPERPOWERS

Transgender role model and pioneer, spotlight sharer.

THEIR INCREDIBLE STORY

An activist for transgender rights and possibly one of the most visible transgender people of recent years, Laverne Cox is an achiever of many firsts as a transgender woman.

Cox rose to prominence thanks to her role in Netflix's *Orange is the New Black* (*OITNB*) as Sophia Burset, an openly transgender character whose storyline did a lot to promote transgender issues and brought these experiences to a wider audience. From this role, Cox began achieving those many firsts, starting with being the first openly transgender person nominated for a Primetime Emmy in the acting category for her role in *OITNB*, and went on to win a Daytime Emmy for her role as executive producer on *Laverne Cox Presents: The T Word*.

Since her time on *OITNB*, Cox has gone on to play a variety of other queer roles, including the legendary Frank-N-Furter in the FX remake of *The Rocky Horror Picture Show*. She also became the first transgender person to portray a transgender character on broadcast television in CBS' *Doubt*.

Prior to her prominence through *OITNB*, Cox was the first transgender person of colour to produce and star in her own show, *TRANSform Me*. Already pioneering transgender visibility, Cox's show saw her team up with two other transgender stylists, Jamie Clayton and Nina Poon, to help makeover a different person each episode. The show was a celebration of transgender identities and forged a connection to the wider community.

Visibility has always been at the centre of Cox's work as an activist for the transgender community, particularly with shows such as *TRANSform Me*, but also with her roles as transgender characters. Cox is, however, always eager to remind others that she doesn't speak to all transgender experiences and that people should seek out conversations and understanding of other queer experiences too.

Thanks to Cox's appearances in fictional and non-fictional media, the conversation on transgender lives and experiences has become more prominent. She takes an active part in the conversations, sharing her experiences and validating the experience of the transgender community as a whole.

"IT IS REVOLUTIONARY FOR ANY TRANS PERSON TO CHOOSE TO BE SEEN AND VISIBLE IN A WORLD THAT TELLS US WE SHOULD NOT EXIST."

THEIR AWESOME ACHIEVEMENTS

→ Became the first openly transgender person to be nominated for a Primetime Emmy in the acting category for her role in *Orange is the New Black*.

→ Won a Daytime Emmy for *Laverne Cox Presents: The T Word* in 2015.

→ Was the first transgender person to portray a transgender character on broadcast television in *Doubt*.

→ Received a Glamour Award for Woman of the Year in 2014.

→ Won the Screen Actors Guild Award for Outstanding Performance by an Ensemble in a Comedy Series for *Orange is the New Black*.

"IF YOU HAVE A PROBLEM WITH PEOPLE LIVING THEIR LIVES AND BEING AUTHENTICALLY WHO THEY ARE, YOU REALLY SHOULD GO AND DO SOME SOUL-SEARCHING."

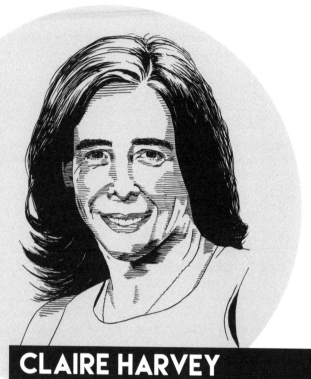

CLAIRE HARVEY

1974–PRESENT

SUPERPOWERS

Paralympian, Role model, LGBTQ activist.

THEIR INCREDIBLE STORY

A pioneer of inclusivity, Claire Harvey is a Paralympic athlete who has represented the UK since 2012 and championed diversity in the UK sports scene.

Harvey's career journey began after an accident in 2008 left her with a paralyzed leg. The incident led to Harvey attending a Paralympic Sports Day to try different activities and eventually she joined the women's national sitting volleyball team. She then went on to focus on track and field athletics, and in 2012 competed in the Paralympics in London. She also competed in the 2015 IPC Athletics World Championships in Berlin, where she came fourth in javelin and eighth in discus. She was unable to compete in the 2016 Paralympics due to an injury.

Harvey initially came out at 15 years old, but with a lack of queer role models she struggled with her identity and tried to fit the brief of how she thought a lesbian should be – at the time a stereotype involving short hair and masculine presentation. Harvey claims to have received a lot of negativity at school from both pupils and teachers for being so open about her sexuality.

Today, Harvey seeks to prevent younger generations suffering because of their sexuality or gender identity. She was appointed chief executive of Diversity Role Models in 2017, an organization that seeks to prevent homophobic, biphobic and transphobic bullying in UK schools by educating young people about LGBTQ walks of life and how the misuse of language can be damaging. Harvey expressed a desire to create a more inclusive culture in schools where young people can be themselves.

In addition to her work in education, Harvey still focuses on inclusivity in sport. She became a patron of Just A Ball Game? – an anti-discrimination organization focused on the sports world. The organization seeks to normalize LGBTQ individuals in sport, as they currently believe the number of publicly out LGBTQ professionals in sport are few and far between. When Harvey became a patron of the organization, she talked about the importance of those who are comfortable being public about their sexuality in sport being visible as role models for young people and showing the diversity of the LGBTQ community.

Harvey's efforts through Diversity Role Models and her platform as a queer Paralympian have given her the chance to be the role model she never had growing up. Her efforts ensure that LGBTQ youth will face less abuse than previous generations and gain a better understanding of queer experiences.

THEIR AWESOME ACHIEVEMENTS

→ Began an athletic career after a paralyzing injury and is now a respected Paralympian.

→ Received the Hero of the Year award at the European Diversity Awards in 2013.

→ Appointed chief executive of Diversity Role Models in 2017.

→ Continues to be a role model to both Paralympians and LGBTQ people worldwide.

→ Shows that it's possible to overcome struggles with identity and go on to do amazing things, including taking an active role in helping those struggling with similar issues.

"YOUNG PEOPLE NEED TO SEE ADULTS AROUND THEM ROLE MODELLING INCLUSIVE BEHAVIOURS. YOU CAN'T BE WHAT YOU DON'T SEE; YOUNG PEOPLE ARE EXCELLENT AT REPLICATING THE ADULTS AROUND THEM."

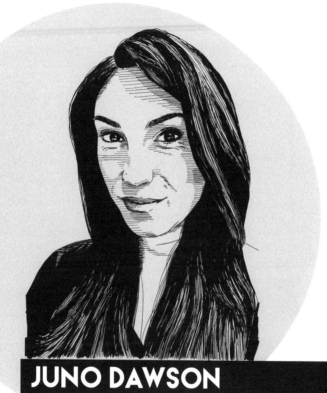

JUNO DAWSON

1981–PRESENT

SUPERPOWERS

Transgender role model, writer, performer, activist.

THEIR INCREDIBLE STORY

British writer and young adult novelist Juno Dawson is known for engendering conversation about LGBTQ rights and experiences, calling for more writers, queer or otherwise, to feature LGBTQ characters to further the visibility of the queer community.

One of Dawson's early books, the groundbreaking *This Book Is Gay*, a guide to growing up LGBTQ written by someone who knows what they're talking about, became the subject of a controversy after its publication in 2014, when residents of Wasilla, Alaska, petitioned to remove it from the local library because of its queer content. Dawson said at the time that the incident highlighted the hatred and prejudice still faced by the LGBTQ community.

Being public about her transition was important to Dawson, as she herself didn't have any transgender role models when growing up. She began to make headlines in 2015 when she came out as transgender, starting with an exclusive Buzzfeed interview where she talked about how she had initially believed she was gay as she had no concept of what transgender identity was. For a while, Dawson accepted the identity of "gay man" though she often felt something was missing or out of reach. She describes the catalyst for starting her own transition as meeting an 11-year-old transgender girl while teaching a writing workshop at a school in London. Dawson admired the young girl's bravery in being her authentic self and it prompted her to begin her transition soon after.

In 2017, Dawson published part-memoir, part gender-theory, *The Gender Games*. The book is considered by academics to be a great starting point for readers on gender theory. In it, Dawson tells her story of growing-up queer and transitioning, sharing her experiences of the expectations of gender forced on her by societal norms and discussing the importance of intersectionality in feminist and queer theory, while always remaining clear that she doesn't speak for the entire transgender community. Dawson was open about experiencing different gender perspectives, and how this gave her experiences of both sides of patriarchal oppression – the construct of gender, as Dawson puts it, isn't just screwing over transgender people, but messing with everyone.

Juno Dawson continues to write for young adults and campaign in the transgender civil rights movement, believing that young people need more queer role models to understand their own experiences. Her books are aimed at younger audiences in order to give them the language and tools to identify as who they are. She isn't afraid to use her own experiences as a means to educate people on transgender experiences and issues, and also to normalize the experiences of those growing up questioning their gender identity. In doing so, Dawson continues to educate on these issues, and gives people going through similar experiences a point of reference to understand themselves (or those around them) a little better.

THEIR AWESOME ACHIEVEMENTS

→ Is a tireless transgender rights activist, writing about transgender issues, creating video campaigns and appearing on talk shows to discuss and defend the transgender community.

→ Has become a public transgender role model calling for more queer and transgender role models and writers.

→ Has written an impressive 14 books to date in a six-year career, with *The Gender Games* soon to become a UK television show. She is unafraid to write about difficult topics in young adult fiction, such as addiction in *Clean* or spine-chilling horror in *Say Her Name.*

→ Won the Queen of Teen award for writing teen fiction in 2014.

"NO PANEL, NO SCIENTIST, NO POLITICIAN, NOT THE WHO, NO ONE CAN TELL ME – OR YOU – HOW IT FEELS TO BE MALE OR FEMALE."

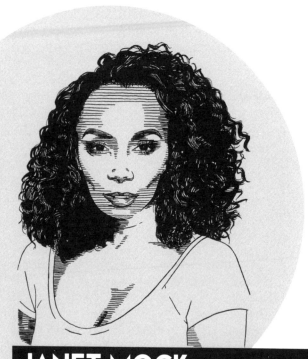

JANET MOCK

1983–PRESENT

SUPERPOWERS

Transgender rights activist, writer, producer, visibility activist.

THEIR INCREDIBLE STORY

Janet Mock graduated from New York University with an MA in journalism in 2006, going on to work for *People* magazine as Staff Editor. Mock made the decision to publicly come out as transgender in a 2011 *Marie Claire* article, putting her in the public spotlight as an advocate for transgender visibility. Right off the bat, Mock began to publicly discuss issues faced by transgender people, starting with the headline given to the *Marie Claire* article – "I was born a boy" – which she did not agree with, as she knew she had always been a girl.

In her 2014 book, *Redefining Realness*, Mock raised the issue again. "I was born into what doctors proclaim is a boy's body. I had no choice in the assignment of my sex at birth... My genital reconstructive surgery did not make me a girl, I was always a girl."

The book furthered the conversation on gender identity and assignment – Mock's perspective being that sex is something assigned to an individual at birth, and that the term "assigned gender" refers to a gender that a transgender person has never identified with.

Instead of distancing herself from *Marie Claire*, Mock became a contributing editor. In her role, Mock publicly discusses transgender issues and transgender representation in the beauty industry.

In 2011, Mock joined the It Gets Better Project, uploading a video of her own experiences as a trans woman, and has been known to start hashtag movements on Twitter, such as #GirlsLikeUs, encouraging transgender women to speak out about their experiences, raising awareness of transgender identities and showing diversity within the transgender community.

Janet Mock has used her high profile to defend other transgender individuals, such as activist Monica Jones who was convicted in 2014 of "manifesting prostitution" in Arizona. Mock has highlighted the ambiguity of the state's discriminatory profiling law in which police have the right to arrest women if they suspect they might be involved in sex work – and where waving at cars or talking to passersby is enough to bring charges against someone. Jones' arrest has been attributed to the "walking while trans" phenomenon, which has seen transgender individuals unfairly targeted by such laws, particularly transgender women of colour.

More recently, Mock wrote and directed an episode of 2018's *Pose*, a drama following the story of New York's ballroom culture of 1987. This makes Mock the first transgender woman of colour to be hired as a writer for a television series and she continues to raise the visibility of the transgender community to this day.

THEIR AWESOME ACHIEVEMENTS

➜ Challenges and changes the understanding of gender and advocates the assigned gender philosophy.

➜ Began transgender visibility campaigns such as #GirlsLikeUs.

➜ Included in the first Trans 100 list recognizing transgender activists, listed in OUT100 Most Compelling People of the Year from *Out Magazine* and featured in *GOOD Magazine*'s GOOD 100 for "building an online army to defend #GirlsLikeUs" in 2013.

➜ Won the Inspiration Award from GLSEN at the Respect Awards and featured in *The Advocate*'s 40 under 40 list in 2014.

➜ Received the Stonewall Book Award from the American Library Association for *Redefining Realness* in 2015.

"LIVING BY OTHER PEOPLE'S DEFINITIONS AND PERCEPTIONS SHRINKS US TO SHELLS OF OURSELVES, RATHER THAN COMPLEX PEOPLE EMBODYING MULTIPLE IDENTITIES."

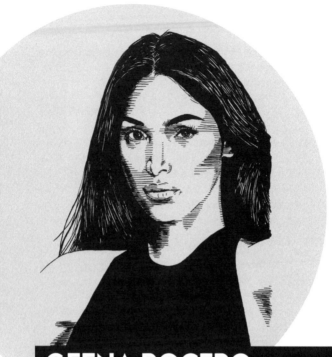

GEENA ROCERO

1983–PRESENT

SUPERPOWERS

Gender Proud founder, transgender rights activist, supermodel.

THEIR INCREDIBLE STORY

Filipino supermodel Geena Rocero is an activist for transgender rights and founder of the Gender Proud organization, who has fought for visibility and to break down barriers for the transgender community.

After moving to New York in 2006, Rocero was discovered in Manhattan by a fashion photographer and spent more than a decade working as a model. It wasn't until 2014 that Rocero would come out as transgender, on International Transgender Day of Visibility.

Rocero came out with a TED talk called "Why I must come out". Acknowledging that she wasn't alone in her experiences, but that she had had a supportive family (something many are not lucky enough to have) who helped her through, Rocero discussed the importance of having transgender role models to look up to.

From a young age, Rocero was fascinated by beauty pageants in the Philippines and she knew she wanted to be like the women who took part in them. She already knew how to self-identify – she knew she was female. A pageant manager helped Rocero join one of the contests when she was 15 years old and she won Best in Swimsuit and Best in Long Gown. For two years Rocero entered beauty pageants, living her truth as a transgender woman.

Rocero's mother, who at the time was living in New York, encouraged her daughter to move to the US.

She told Rocero that in the US she would legally be able to change her gender marker and name in line with her identity. However, Rocero discovered that in the US it was only possible to make these legal changes after undergoing gender-confirmation surgery. Rocero's supportive mother joined her on a journey to Thailand, where Rocero underwent surgery to alter her body. Upon returning to the US, Rocero moved to San Francisco and was granted a driver's licence under the name Geena with the gender marker F.

Since coming out as transgender, Rocero has founded Gender Proud, a two-part organization that advocates for transgender rights and runs a production studio of transgender media. The production side, which has a focus on visibility, has created series such as *Beautiful as I Want to Be*, *Willing & Able* and *No League of Their Own*, each focusing on a different aspect of transgender experiences. As an advocacy organization, Gender Proud focuses on breaking down the barriers faced by transgender people and empowering communities globally to advocate for their legal rights.

Rocero still focuses her efforts on the visibility of transgender lives, and continues to model and fight for the rights of transgender people both in the USA and worldwide.

THEIR AWESOME ACHIEVEMENTS

→ Won pageants and went on to become a supermodel in the US.

→ Came out publicly in a TED talk and acknowledged the necessity for transgender role models.

→ Founded the Gender Proud organization, which continues to share transgender experiences and fight for transgender equality worldwide.

→ Elected to the LGBT Community Centre Board in New York City.

→ Continues to tirelessly raise transgender visibility both locally and worldwide.

"THE WORLD MAKES YOU SOMETHING THAT YOU'RE NOT – BUT YOU KNOW INSIDE WHAT YOU ARE."

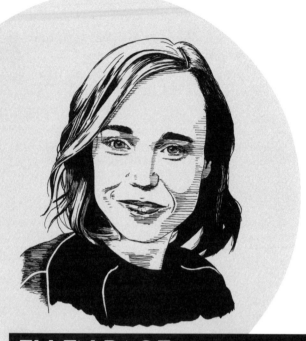

ELLEN PAGE

1987–PRESENT

SUPERPOWERS

Award-winning actress, activist, pro-choice feminist, out and proud lesbian, wearer of amazing suits.

THEIR INCREDIBLE STORY

Ellen Page, the actress from *Juno* who warmed hearts and empowered young people worldwide with an incredibly sincere coming out speech, boasts both a diverse list of film roles and an impressive suit collection.

Page became an instant LGBTQ icon in 2014, on Valentine's Day no less, at the Time to Thrive conference hosted by the Human Rights Campaign, with an open, honest and touching coming out speech. Page told everyone how she hoped her coming out would make a difference to those still in the closet, struggling to come out themselves, and give them an easier time. "I am tired of hiding and I am tired of lying by omission," were Page's defiant words shortly after announcing her sexuality, to a standing ovation.

As with anyone famous, the act of coming out alone is empowering. Page's coming out was something more than that. Being so young herself, she showed a level of understanding and empathy with young queers across the world – people who might be struggling to come out to their parents or friends. The applause from the audience that day wasn't just congratulatory, or a celebration of Page's bravery, but also a thank you for empowering people struggling everywhere.

Page's speech also presented a perfect opportunity to speak about gender, and specifically, the gender stereotyping and crushing standards forced upon actors by the film industry and tabloids. When a tabloid reporter asked Page why she chose to dress like a "massive man", her response was a defiant: "Because I like to be comfortable." Perhaps also in defiance, since her coming out speech, Page has been known to wear some very stylish, sharp-looking suits.

Soon after her Time to Thrive speech, Page co-produced and starred in *Freeheld* in her first LGBTQ role, portraying the true story of Stacie Andree, partner of Laurel Hester. Based on a documentary of the same name, *Freeheld* depicts Hester's battle with terminal cancer, as well as her struggles with the Ocean County, New Jersey, Board of Chosen Freeholders to have her pension benefits transferred to her domestic partner, Andree. The role was seen as symbolic of Page's recent coming out and an acceptance of her identity and true self.

In addition to taking on queer film roles, Page is an active, vocal and most importantly visible member of the LGBTQ community. Particularly on social media, Page often discusses LGBTQ rights and how important it is to remember the struggles faced by the community.

THEIR AWESOME ACHIEVEMENTS

➜ Empowered a generation of queer people with a sincere coming out speech.

➜ Encouraged and empowered a generation to feel comfortable in their bodies and their gender in the same speech.

➜ Appeared in *The Advocate*'s 40 under 40 list – featuring inspiring people under 40 with an important message for all generations.

➜ Won numerous film awards, including Best Actress for *Juno* from many awarding bodies.

➜ Nominated for Academy Awards, BAFTAs, Golden Globes and Screen Actors Guild Awards for *Juno*.

"WHEN WE'RE GROWING UP THERE ARE ALL SORTS OF PEOPLE TELLING US WHAT TO DO WHEN REALLY WHAT WE NEED IS SPACE TO WORK OUT WHO TO BE."

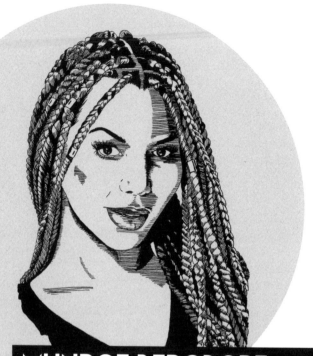

MUNROE BERGDORF

1987–PRESENT

SUPERPOWERS

Transgender model, equal and civil rights activist, diversity advocate.

THEIR INCREDIBLE STORY

Munroe Bergdorf made waves as L'Oréal's first openly transgender model in 2017. She later become known for a controversy surrounding comments she made on racism, but would become iconic for the way she stood her ground during the incident. However, Bergdorf's work as an LGBTQ activist, particularly for transgender women of colour, is often overlooked.

While studying at the University of Brighton, Bergdorf began to identify as genderqueer. After graduating she became involved in fashion PR and began transitioning. During her transition, she became involved in fashion modelling and made it clear she wanted to change the lack of transgender visibility on the catwalk. By being a visible transwoman, Bergdorf saw a means to diversify the industry.

Bergdorf's L'Oréal campaign, which focused on diversity, gave her an amazing opportunity to reach and empower people with similar experiences to her own, and to show the world that transgender is beautiful. Sadly, due to the aforementioned online controversy, Bergdorf was only briefly involved in the campaign.

In 2017, the Unite the Right Rally in Charlottesville US saw white supremacists clash with protestors. Seeing the violence of this far right group, Bergdorf felt she could not hold her silence. She wrote a

Facebook post acknowledging that she had very little energy remaining to cope with all this violence. However, she went on to say that a system of oppression had been built by white people, a violent system built on the backs of people of colour and this violence was the result of that system. She said this system benefited all white people, and that they needed to admit to this in order to begin to make meaningful change.

The comments were picked up by the British press and L'Oréal let Bergdorf go. Bergdorf then elaborated on her comments, which had largely been twisted by the media to imply she was saying all white people were racist and ignorant. She clarified that racism is a social structure that cannot be brought down by any individual, but must be dismantled by the society that built it and not doing anything to challenge that system would make someone complicit in it.

She bounced back from the controversies, temporarily joining the UK's Labour Party as LGBTQ advisor and being hired as a model to front a campaign for cruelty-free cosmetic brand Illamasqua, which celebrated her individuality and embodiment of diversity. Illamasqua also stood by Bergdorf's comments on racism, accepting that they had been taken out of context by the media.

THEIR AWESOME ACHIEVEMENTS

→ Became the first transgender person to front a beauty campaign for L'Oréal.

→ Held a post as LGBTQ advisor to the UK's Labour Party.

→ Hired to front Illamasqua Beauty Spotlight campaign focusing on gender fluidity in 2017.

→ Used her platform to raise awareness of institutional racism despite risks to her reputation and career.

→ Continues to push conversations on race and gender on her blog.

"THE WORLD IS SO DIVIDED BUT, WHEN WE THINK ABOUT EQUALITY, WE NEED TO BE THINKING IN A WORLDWIDE SENSE. WE ARE ALL HUMAN BEINGS."

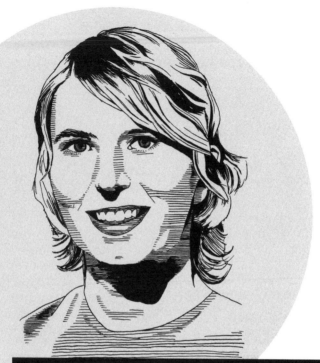

CHELSEA MANNING

1987–PRESENT

SUPERPOWERS

Whistleblower, indomitable transgender activist.

THEIR INCREDIBLE STORY

As a whistleblower, the reasons behind Chelsea Manning's fame are somewhat controversial. However, her humanitarian beliefs are unquestionable, and her visibility as a transgender person and speaking on LGBTQ issues makes her a queer icon.

Most were unaware of Manning until 2010 when she was charged for leaking sensitive and classified information on the Iraq War to WikiLeaks. She also leaked documents on other secretive activities of questionable efforts by the US Army and Government, due to her strong opposition to these practices.

No one can say Manning didn't have conviction – the leak initially put her at risk of a death sentence, however this was later shortened to 35 years in prison. Seven years later, President Barack Obama commuted all but four months of Manning's sentence. She was not pardoned, but Obama believed that the sentence had been too severe. Manning was released later in 2017, having served four years.

Manning began to experience gender dysmorphia while serving in the army and in 2009 contacted a gender counsellor. However, due to the US army's "Don't ask, don't tell" policy on sexuality, Manning felt isolated and depressed. Poor working conditions also contributed to her depression and emotional instability. Many anti-LGBTQ groups used this instability to protest against LGBTQ individuals serving in the military. However, in a positive twist Manning's story shone a light on the damage that the "Don't ask, don't tell" policy could inflict and the poor treatment of LGBTQ individuals, particularly transgender people, in the military. While Manning has never officially been linked to the ending of "Don't ask, don't tell", she has spoken out against it and her story possibly contributed to the decision to repeal in 2011.

Manning struggled to adapt to life outside prison, saying that the world had already changed drastically in those four years. She has expressed her fears about the political climate and attitudes toward marginalized groups, such as the LGBTQ community, and still campaigns for positive change for the LGBTQ community, particularly those serving in the military. She has spoken out in particular against recent government policy that bans transgender people serving in the US military. Manning was brave enough to attend the Pride celebrations in New York City almost immediately after her release, where she represented the American Civil Liberties Union.

THEIR AWESOME ACHIEVEMENTS

→ Blew the whistle on atrocities, collateral damage and non-ethical action undertaken by the US Army and Government.

→ Highlighted the poor treatment of transgender people and the LGBTQ community as a whole within the military.

→ Spoke out against the military's "Don't ask, don't tell" policy, which was repealed in 2011.

→ Continues to fight for government transparency and LGBTQ rights in spite of fears and threats to her safety.

"THE PAST WILL ALWAYS AFFECT ME, AND I WILL KEEP THAT IN MIND WHILE REMEMBERING THAT HOW IT PLAYED OUT IS ONLY MY STARTING POINT, NOT MY FINAL DESTINATION."

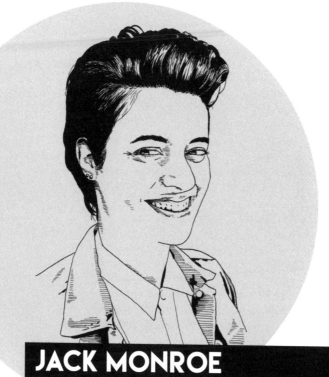

JACK MONROE

1988–PRESENT

SUPERPOWERS

Non-binary role model, poverty survivor, anti-austerity campaigner, food educator.

THEIR INCREDIBLE STORY

Food blogger and British poverty campaigner Jack Monroe is well known for speaking out against the UK government and its austerity policies. Monroe identifies as non-binary (and has also identified as a transgender non-binary woman) and has talked publicly about gender identity and LGBTQ issues.

Monroe comes from a working-class background and didn't pursue academia, instead working locally in a chip shop and for the Essex County Fire and Rescue service. After having a child, Monroe fell into poverty, being unable to arrange work around childcare responsibilities. Financial hardship led to Monroe writing the blog A Girl Called Jack, which saw the publication of simple and interesting recipes people could cook on a very tight food budget – with Monroe looking to the UK supermarkets' cheapest own-brand ranges for inspiration. Around this time Monroe chose the name Jack, a nickname short for "Jack of all trades". When Monroe came out publicly as non-binary, the blog was renamed Cooking on a Bootstrap.

Monroe's blog quickly gained traction, with many parents who struggled to make ends meet turning to the cheap-and-easy-to-make recipes within. This helped to bring Monroe to a wider audience and to become established as a writer – later becoming a columnist for *The Echo* and for *The Huffington Post*, further increasing Monroe's public profile.

With this rise in online fame, Monroe was one of four food-loving bloggers to be approached by Sainsbury's to be the face of their 2013 marketing campaign. Monroe had turned down similar offers from other supermarkets such as Waitrose, saying that it felt right to accept Sainsbury's offer due to the chain's ethical policies. There was no questioning Monroe's charitability or humility either – rather than accepting the whole fee for the campaign, Monroe accepted the equivalent of the living wage, and requested that the remaining budget be donated to local charities and food banks, to better help those struggling in poverty.

Poverty has always been an issue close to Monroe's heart, due to past experiences struggling to make ends meet. Monroe has campaigned for a number of charitable causes since rising to fame, particularly those that seek to end child poverty, such as Oxfam, Child Poverty Action and The Trussell Trust.

On National Coming Out Day in 2015, Monroe publicly came out as non-binary transgender, emphasizing that not all transgender people transition from one binary gender to another. However, when Monroe's story was told by the *Daily Mail*, the British tabloid linked Monroe's coming out to a break up with their partner at the time, and made several intrusive comments about Monroe's body and claimed that "Jack" was not Monroe's "real" name. Monroe publicly called out the *Daily*

Mail, fighting against media insensitivity around transgender lives and their portrayal. Monroe continues to campaign against poverty and austerity in the UK and fights for queer visibility.

THEIR AWESOME ACHIEVEMENTS

→ Awarded an MBE in 2007 for services to children and families.

→ Received an honorary degree from the University of Essex in 2015.

→ Awarded Woman of the Future Award after coming out as transgender in 2015 (Monroe also identifies as non-binary).

→ Became a patron of The Food Chain, food blog and organization fighting against HIV and providing nutritional advice to those with HIV.

→ Continues to vocally campaign against the British government's austerity measures and the poverty those measures force people into.

→ Speaks out for the LGBTQ community, particularly on transgender issues.

"I WANT TO BE TREATED AS A PERSON, NOT AS A WOMAN OR A MAN."

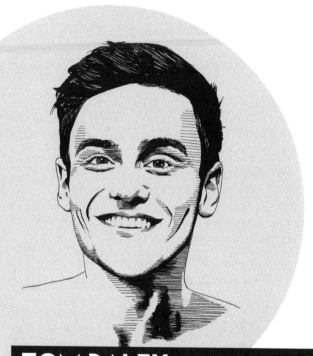

TOM DALEY

1994–PRESENT

SUPERPOWERS

Olympic diver and swimmer, gold medal winner, LGBTQ visibility activist.

THEIR INCREDIBLE STORY

Olympic diver, gold medal winner and LGBTQ activist Tom Daley is well known for his record-breaking athletic achievements. He's also well known for his public coming out and subsequent LGBTQ visibility activism.

Daley came to prominence early in life thanks to his diving prowess. From the age of nine he was making waves in both national and international competitions, and in 2008 at the age of 14, became the youngest person to represent Britain in the Olympics and the youngest person from any nation to participate in the final. Daley has continued to break records ever since.

In 2013, Daley came out publicly in a YouTube video. In the video Daley said he had been in relationships with women in the past, but now he was in a relationship with a man and he had never been happier. Initially he wanted to keep his relationship private, but eventually he revealed his partner to be screenwriter Dustin Lance Black. Since coming out Daley has been non-specific on his identity, though more recently he has said he identifies as queer.

Daley and Black announced their engagement in 2015 and were married two years later. Their first child (via a surrogate) was born in 2018. Sadly, this final announcement caused almost immediate criticisms from anti-LGBTQ groups and individuals. However, many also spoke out to support and congratulate the couple, which could perhaps be a positive indication that attitudes toward LGBTQ families are changing for the better.

Social media has been more than a platform for Daley to come out. The act itself was empowering for the young LGBTQ community and Daley often posts videos about his life with Black, normalizing queer lives for Daley's many followers and fans.

In 2015, Daley became a patron for the LGBTQ charity Switchboard. The charity formed in the 1970s – providing support and information to London's gay community after the decriminalization of homosexuality in 1967 – and became the leading source of information during the HIV/AIDS crisis of the 1980s. Daley helped the charity rebrand to be as inclusive as possible, now providing support to the whole LGBTQ community.

Daley continues to be a voice of the LGBTQ community, sharing his experiences with a wide audience and normalizing queer experiences, while also forging ahead with his successful career as a diver.

THEIR AWESOME ACHIEVEMENTS

→ Publicly came out and has discussed his queer identity, giving visibility and voice to the LGBTQ community.

→ Supports LGBTQ charities such as Switchboard.

→ Received The Herald Awards Sports Personality of the Year in 2007, 2008 and 2012.

→ Winner of BBC Young Sports Personality of the Year in 2008 and 2010.

→ Awarded Best Sports Star at BBC Radio 1's Teen Awards in 2010, Best Young Sports Star in 2011 and Best British Sports Star in 2012.

→ Received Independent Influencer Award at the British LGBT Awards in 2017.

"MY LGBT HERO IS ANYONE THAT IS BRAVE ENOUGH TO BE WHO THEY ARE, AND EMBRACE IT, AND BE PROUD OF IT – BECAUSE PEOPLE LIKE THAT ARE ABLE TO ENCOURAGE OTHER PEOPLE TO DO THE SAME."

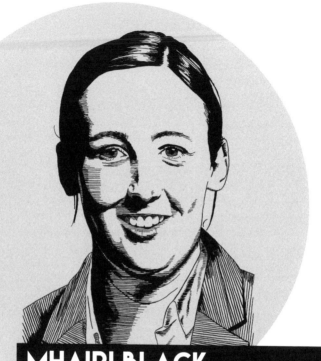

MHAIRI BLACK

1994–PRESENT

SUPERPOWERS

*UK's youngest politician, out and proud,
no-nonsense political speaker.*

THEIR INCREDIBLE STORY

Mhairi Black is a Scottish MP well known for her attitudes toward British politics, often critical of the government's approach to poverty and unemployment – something she made clear in her maiden speech as an MP. Her extremely impassioned and quotable speeches have made her a popular sight on social media feeds, making her a particular hit with younger voters. Her queer identity has also made her popular with LGBTQ voters.

Black became the UK's youngest elected MP since at least 1832 when she was elected to the Scottish National Party in 2015 at the age of 20. Her maiden speech garnered millions of online viewings. In it, Black criticized the government for removing housing benefits for people under 21 years of age: a policy that put many young people at risk of homelessness or of being stuck in an abusive environment, as well as generally restricting the freedom of young people. Black pointed out the ridiculousness that as an MP she was then the only 20-year-old in the country able to claim assistance with housing, saying: "Because I am an MP, not only am I the youngest, but I am also the only 20-year-old in the whole of the UK that the chancellor is prepared to help with housing."

Thanks to her impassioned speeches, critical of a government that caused so much poverty in the UK (particularly her home country of Scotland), Black proved popular enough to be re-elected in 2017. Since her election, she has stood vocally against the Conservative government's austerity policies, which have forced many into poverty.

In 2017, Black called out the hypocrisy of a Conservative ruling party that had forced the country into austerity, but after a snap election had to prop up their government by securing a £1 billion deal with Northern Ireland's Democratic Unionist Party (which has a strong anti-LGBTQ stance). This came at a similar time when the pension age for women had been changed without proper warning, with Black further questioning why the government was unable to support their citizens – "pensions are not a benefit, they are a right". In the same speech, Black questioned why the government could always find money for causes like war, but struggled to ensure constituents did not fall into poverty.

Black is openly lesbian and has never made a secret of this fact. When asked about the pressures of coming out, Black responded, "I've never been in." As a supporter of LGBTQ rights, Black has publicly called out the British press for its scathing and perpetual attack of the transgender community. She says that the "trans hysteria" of the media undermines gender recognition progress and laws.

Black remains the youngest member of UK Parliament, and continues to be one of the most vocal on poverty and LGBTQ rights.

THEIR AWESOME ACHIEVEMENTS

→ Appeared on Young Women's Movement Scotland 30 under 30 list.

→ Became the youngest member of UK Parliament – at the age of 20 – since at least the Reform Act of 1832.

→ Became a role model to inspire young people, particularly the young LGBTQ community, to take an interest and get involved in politics.

→ Proudly defended LGBTQ people in politics.

"LET US COME TOGETHER, LET US BE THAT OPPOSITION, LET US BE THAT SIGNPOST OF A BETTER SOCIETY. ULTIMATELY PEOPLE ARE NEEDING A VOICE, PEOPLE ARE NEEDING HELP, LET'S GIVE THEM IT."

READING LIST

From Ace to Ze by
Harriet Dyer

Transgender History
by Susan Stryker

Queer: A Graphic History
by Meg-John Barker

From Prejudice to Pride:
A History of LGBTQ+
Movement by Amy Lamé

It's Okay to be Gay: Celebrity
Coming Out Stories by Val
McDermid, Evan Davis et al

The Harvey Milk Interviews:
In His Own Words by Harvey
Milk, edited by Vince Emery

I Have Chosen to Stay and
Fight by Margaret Cho

Love, Ellen by Betty
DeGeneres

Redefining Realness
by Janet Mock

To The Stars: The
Autobiography by
George Takei

Daring to be Myself: A
Memoir by Laverne Cox

My Life by Marlene Dietrich

Not My Father's Son
by Alan Cumming

Moab is My Washpot
by Stephen Fry

Doll Parts by Amanda Lepore

Stone Butch Blues by
Leslie Feinberg

Lettin It All Hang
Out by RuPaul

Freddie Mercury: His
Life in His Own Words
by Greg Brooks, edited
by Simon Lupton

Man into Woman: The First
Sex Change by Lili Elbe,
edited by Niels Hoyer

Lou Sullivan: Daring to
be a Man Amongst Men
by Dr Brice D. Smith

A Burst of Light and Other
Essays by Audre Lorde

I Am Your Sister by
Audre Lorde

The Cancer Journals
by Audre Lorde

Tipping the Velvet
by Sarah Waters

Oranges Are Not the Only
Fruit by Jeanette Winterson

The Gender Games: The
Problem with Men and
Women from Someone
Who Has Been Both
by Juno Dawson

WATCH LIST

The films below can be found across various platforms, some are biographical and some fictionalized works based on real experiences. Some are educational and informative on the queer experience, and some are groundbreaking in their content or even their casting.

Milk (film, 2008)

Laverne Cox Presents: The T Word (documentary, 2014)

Stephen Fry: Out There (documentary, 2013)

To Be Takei (documentary, 2014)

Party Monster: The Shockumentary (documentary, 1998)

The Death and Life of Marsha P. Johnson (documentary, 2017)

Stormé: The Lady of the Jewel Box (short film, 1987)

Battle of the Sexes (film, 2017)

Geena Rocero: Why I Must Come Out (TED talk, 2014)

Happy Birthday, Marsha! (short film, 2016)

Outlaw (documentary, 1994 – search online for Leslie Feinberg on Discovering Transgender History)

Lou Sullivan on Honesty and AIDS: 1988–1990 (Youtube clip, 2010)

Audre Lorde – The Berlin Years 1984–1992 (documentary, 2012)

Pose (television series, 2018)

Gaycation (television series, 2016)

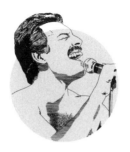

Have you enjoyed this book?
If so, why not write a review on
your favourite website?

If you're interested in finding out more
about our books, find us on Facebook
at **Summersdale Publishers** and follow
us on Twitter at **@Summersdale.**

Thanks very much for buying
this Summersdale book.

www.summersdale.com